Winning *with* Diabetes

Inspiring stories of famous and not-so-famous people with diabetes who live life abundantly.

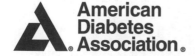

American Diabetes Association®

PRODUCTION DIRECTOR
Carolyn R. Segree

PRODUCTION COORDINATOR
Peggy M. Rote

BOOK DESIGN
Wickham & Associates, Inc.

TYPESETTING SERVICES
James Stein Communications

EDITOR
Sherrye Landrum

PRINTED IN CANADA

1 3 5 7 9 10 8 6 4 2

The suggestions and information contained in this publication are generally consistent with the Clinical Practice Recommendations and other policies of the American Diabetes Association, but they do not represent the policy or position of the Association or any of its boards or committees. Reasonable steps have been taken to ensure the accuracy of the information presented. However, the American Diabetes Association cannot ensure the safety or efficacy of any product or service described in this publication. Individuals are advised to consult a physician or other appropriate health care professional before undertaking any diet or exercise program or taking any medication referred to in this publication. Professionals must use and apply their own professional judgment, experience, and training and should not rely solely on the information contained in this publication before prescribing any diet, exercise, or medication. The American Diabetes Association—its officers, directors, employees, volunteers, and members—assumes no responsibility or liability for personal or other injury, loss, or damage that may result from the suggestions or information in this publication.

AMERICAN DIABETES ASSOCIATION
1660 DUKE STREET
ALEXANDRIA, VIRGINIA 22314

Library of Congress Cataloging-in-Publication Data

Winning with diabetes : inspiring stories of famous and not-so-famous people with diabetes
    who live life abundantly / American Diabetes Association.
        p.   cm.
    ISBN 0-945448-97-X (pbk.)
    1. Diabetics--United States--Biography. 2. Celebrities--United States--Biography.
I. American Diabetes Association.
RC660.4.W56   1998
362.1'96462'00922--dc21
    [B]   97-49112
                                                                        CIP

Contents

Foreword

Do you ever visualize diabetes as your opponent in a competitive game? It may seem strange, but in many ways, this analogy holds truer than many people would like to believe. In fact, all of the people in this book from the American Diabetes Association have won or excelled not only at what they do for their livelihood, but in their ability to compete with diabetes. And I mean that in both senses—they "compete" while having diabetes, and they compete against the opponent diabetes. Each one has been featured on the cover of *Diabetes Forecast* magazine and is "famous" for their unique "game strategy." Their *Forecast* success stories are gathered here.

Vince Lombardi's dictum was: "The quality of a person's life is in direct proportion to their commitment to excellence, regardless of their chosen field of endeavor." We have profiled professional athletes with diabetes such as my all-time favorite hockey player Bobby Clarke, tennis star Bill Talbert, and football player Art Shell. They have been intense competitors in their sports as well as in dealing with diabetes—battling diabetes as hard as they battled their sporting opponents. But it isn't just the athletes who have followed Lombardi's declaration that "Winning is a habit. Unfortunately, so is losing. If you can accept losing, you can't win." We also profile people famous in print, television, and music. Others are famous for humanitarian work or living rich, full lives. Each person in this book has lost occasional games or tournaments, but never the whole season or their commitment to beat diabetes. In every case, you'll read about a winner.

I have always objected to the term "diabetic" when it is used as a noun to describe a person. To me, this implies that the person has given up the competition and is merely trying to appease his opponent. It reminds me of what

Winston Churchill said, "An appeaser is one who feeds a crocodile, hoping it will eat him last." No one in this book will ever consider that an option in their contest with diabetes. Each one has made contributions to our lives and provided examples to show us how to play the game well against an able opponent.

Neil Friedman, MD
Editor-in-Chief
Diabetes Forecast

Acknowledgments

Samuel L. Abbate, MD, CDE
Marshfield Clinic
Marshfield, Wisconsin

Eva Brzezinski, RD, MS
The University of California at San Diego Medical Center
San Diego, California

Connie C. Crawley, RD, BS, MS
The University of Georgia Cooperative Extension Service
Athens, Georgia

John T. Devlin, MD
Maine Medical Center
Portland, Maine

Alan M. Jacobson, MD
Joslin Diabetes Center
Boston, Massachusetts

Lois Jovanovic-Peterson, MD
Sansum Medical Research Foundation
Santa Barbara, California

Carolyn Leontos, MS, RD, CDE
The University of Nevada Cooperative Extension
Las Vegas, Nevada

Peter A. Lodewick, MD
Diabetes Care Center
Birmingham, Alabama

Carol E. Malcom, BSN, CDE
Seattle, Washington

Wylie McNabb, EdD
The University of Chicago Center for Medical Education
and Health Care
Chicago, Illinois

Virginia Peragallo-Dittko, RN, MA, CDE
Winthrop University Hospital
Mineola, New York

Jacqueline Siegel, RN
St. Joseph Hospital
Seattle, Washington

Tim Wysocki, PhD
Nemours Children's Clinic
Jacksonville, Florida

Robert M. Anderson, EdD
Michigan Diabetes Research and Training Center
The University of Michigan Medical School
Ann Arbor, Michigan

Janine C. Freeman, RD, CDE
Georgia Center for Diabetes at Columbia Dunwoody
Medical Center
Atlanta, Georgia

Glimmers on the Silver Screen

by Holly Burnett

This article appeared in *Diabetes Forecast,* February 1996.

Imagine Norma Desmond descending her grand Sunset Boulevard staircase and pausing on the last step to utter, "Mr. DeMille, I'm ready for my insulin."

The awareness we might have had.

Paige was born with only one kidney. When we met in college, I was struck by her Lucille Ball–red hair, her devious sense of humor, and her constant trips to the bathroom. She joined in when we all joked about her pea-size bladder, and friends discussed whose kidney she'd take (if she ever needed one), as if it were an honor of friendship, like being selected as a bridesmaid in her wedding. Paige loved children, and after college she accepted a long-term au pair position with a prestigious Southern family.

On one of her visits in 1989, we went to see the newly released film version of *Steel Magnolias.* The story of a group of strong Southern women seemed an ideal choice for us, born and educated as we were south of the Mason-Dixon Line.

The film opens on the fictional little town of Chinquapin, Louisiana, which is abuzz in preparation for the wedding of Shelby Eatenton, played by wholesomely beautiful Julia Roberts in only her second starring role. (She received an Academy Award nomination and a Golden Globe Award for her performance.)

The female characters are introduced as they congregate at Truvy's beauty parlor, no more than a room with a back porch attached to Truvy's house. As the women are being coiffed in preparation for the wedding, Shelby begins to shake violently. The women rush to her aid with orange juice as the audience learns that Shelby has diabetes, kidney problems, and has been told she shouldn't have children.

Against everyone's wishes, Shelby becomes pregnant. "I would rather have 30 minutes of wonderful," she says, "than a lifetime of nothing special." Shelby gives birth to a baby boy, and, after an unsuccessful kidney transplant, dies.

The audience wept quietly, but Paige was crying as if she had lost her own child. In the car, Paige told me that she had just recently been diagnosed with diabetes.

Uncommon Or Common?

Steel Magnolias scared Paige and many other women because it showed a worst-case scenario and promoted the idea that women with diabetes can't have children. Today, in light of improved care for women with diabetes and new drugs to delay, and possibly prevent, kidney disease, Shelby's experience has become the exception. Paige knows this now. Her diabetes is very well controlled. She's healthy and attending graduate school in Chicago.

Admittedly, most of my medical knowledge has come to me subliminally through motion pictures, and I depend on screenwriters to accurately tell the facts. But no one can blame *Steel Magnolias* playwright and screenwriter Robert Harling. His story wasn't meant to be about every woman with diabetes contemplating a pregnancy. His was about one woman: his sister, Susan, who died of diabetes complications in 1985. Harling depicted his family's tragedy in the context of a loyal circle of friends and the Louisiana lifestyle. It's this interweaving of plot and personality that distinguishes *Steel Magnolias* and keeps it from becoming a "Peyton Place with Diabetes."

Three years earlier, in 1986, Rick Podell and Michael Preminger's box office success, *Nothing in Common,* broke significant ground, in terms of diabetes. This comedy-drama focuses on up-and-coming advertising executive David Basner (portrayed by Tom Hanks). Basner juggles a career, the impending divorce of his parents, and the painful realization that his father, Max, has suffered from undiagnosed diabetes for several years.

Gregarious Max Basner is based on screenwriter Rick Podell's own father, David. Max (brilliantly portrayed by Jackie Gleason in one of his finest dramatic performances) is a drinking, cigar-smoking womanizer. His wife Lorraine (Eva Marie Saint), who married Max right out of Catholic school, dismisses her marriage to Max as nothing more than having had a roommate for 34 years. Son David is left to play referee and pseudo-parent to Lorraine and Max, who, without each other, have difficulty coping with daily life.

David has only an impatient tolerance for his father; he's convinced they have nothing in common. But there are obvious parallels between David and Max. David is sexually and socially indulgent. But he's got some of his mother in him, too. He's aware that he must settle into a monogamous relationship to have the type of home Max didn't provide.

After Max smashes his car into a Chicago city bus, David arranges an appointment for him with an eye doctor. Knowing he's ill, Max avoids it, choosing instead to stay planted in his easy chair where he can peacefully drink, smoke, and listen to jazz.

When David helps his father with his slippers one night, he is shocked to see Max's toes have turned black from gangrene. Kicking and cursing, Max is dragged to the hospital where he is diagnosed with diabetes and must have his toes and part of one foot amputated.

A major misconception about diabetes surfaces when Lorraine says to David, "You don't die from diabetes." But David answers, "You do if you let it go this long, Mom! It's the number three cause of death in the country; number one cause of new blindness." (Note: Now diabetes is the fourth leading cause of death by disease.)

This unfortunate scenario is far more common than the one in *Steel Magnolias*. It illustrates the importance of awareness and education in our society, and the great role that denial and fear play in many undiagnosed diabetes cases.

Little Black Bag

Nothing in Common and *Steel Magnolias* were commercial successes that accurately depicted diabetes. But ask people to name a movie about diabetes, and many would say

Reversal of Fortune. They know the 1990 movie is about the court case of Claus Von Bulow, who was accused of injecting his wife, Martha "Sunny" Von Bulow, with insulin in an attempt to kill her. She is still in a coma today.

With the media circus Von Bulow attracted, millions of Americans sat glued to live CNN trial coverage. Some mistakenly concluded that Sunny had diabetes and that Claus tried to kill his wife with the same medication she would have needed to sustain her life.

In the film Alan Dershowitz (played by Ron Silver), Von Bulow's legal counsel at the appeal, seeks to discredit the state of Rhode Island's medical testimony against his client. With only 45 days to file an appeal, Dershowitz enlists the help of his best law students to tear apart the state's case.

Enter Von Bulow, an emotionally restrained British aristocrat with a pallor reminiscent of a mortician's best work. He is a man who would prefer to sit quietly eating his ginger prawns, but he must defend himself at numerous meetings with Dershowitz's team, who have concluded that he is most likely guilty of something.

His attempts at humor don't help him, such as when he quips, "What do you give a wife who has everything? An injection of insulin." At such times, he certainly appears to be the monster the prosecution had described. (Jeremy Irons played the imperious Von Bulow and won an Academy Award for Best Actor.)

Dershowitz successfully discredited the state's testimony that an insulin-encrusted needle had been found in the infamous "little black bag."

A Little More Exposure

Law and diabetes are also explored within the storyline of the 1991 drama *Regarding Henry*. An elderly gentleman, Mr. Matthews, claims he told an admitting nurse he had diabetes but was given the wrong medication. Hot-shot attorney Henry Turner (played by Harrison Ford) represents the hospital and wins the case, alleging Matthews is an alcoholic who probably doesn't know what he said to the admitting nurse.

After Turner is shot in the head during a robbery, he suffers brain damage and must re-learn basic motor and emotional skills. He develops a new perspective on life. He discovers that he and his law firm withheld a witness's testimony stating that Mr. Matthews did indeed inform the admitting nurse that he had diabetes, but the nurse neglected to write it on his chart. Turner delivers the withheld testimony to Mr. Matthews so that he can successfully sue the hospital.

While diabetes is a small part of *Regarding Henry,* it is significant because it again provides exposure, awareness, and education.

Not all references to diabetes are accurate, however, even in the 1990s. In the action-adventure *Cliffhanger* (1993), the bad guys try to convince the Rocky Mountain Rescue Team to help them after their plane has crash-landed. Over the radio, the pilot sends the false message, "Billy's going into shock. We need insulin."

The voice sounded panicky enough to convince the rescuers that this was no ruse. Team members played by Sylvester Stallone and Janine Turner head up the mountain in a blizzard. But a person in shock needs glucose, not insulin.

If art imitates life, then Hollywood has a lot of catching up to do. It has denied diabetes its significance until recently. Had a handful of the great screen classics intertwined their plots with diabetes, the greater awareness of this disease might have saved, or improved, innumerable lives.

Holly Burnett works at ADA and is a film historian, film teacher, and freelance writer.

Gordon Jump: Gotta Act

by Marie McCarren

This article appeared in *Diabetes Forecast,* August 1994.

Mention Mr. Carlson of *WKRP in Cincinnati* at a party and someone's bound to say, "God as my witness…" and more than likely someone else will finish it: "I thought turkeys could fly." Then people will laugh so hard that even those who didn't see the show will start to smile at the fictional radio station's ill-conceived Thanksgiving Day promotion (live turkeys dropped from a helicopter).

Gordon Jump, who played station manager Mr. Carlson, would consider that reaction proof of a job well done. "I hope I give people a chance to laugh. To me that's what it's all about—for people to think about something other than their daily problems."

But suspense can be as much fun as comedy. Lest you think Jump wants you to spend all your free time laughing, you may see him in the mystery-thriller *Bitter Vengeance* filmed for the USA Network (on cable TV). Jump has "not a large role, but a nice, working-actor's role." And, again, it fulfills what he sees as his responsibility to his craft.

"I don't think there's anything more thrilling than touching an audience with information that will make them laugh, or think, or cry," he says.

But shock, horror, despair…he'll leave the creation of those emotions to others—to the makers of what he describes as "garbage."

"I think any television piece that leaves an image of violence or emotional distress influences the actions of the people who watch that show," he says. "What we feed the subconscious—as we're sitting in the theater, reading a book, or looking at a magazine—is going to have some effect upon our actions later."

Yeah, but whose fault is that? People must be asking for it.

"People don't demand that," he insists. "No one demands to regress." No, Jump lays the blame squarely on the shoulders of the garbage-makers.

"Media can be used in either a positive or negative way," he says. "Right now, because it's so money-oriented, we've lost a sense of responsibility to the craft. Greed has become a tremendous driving force in media. Television, film, newspaper, magazine—they do anything that will sell for a buck. When money is the only motivating factor, then you've done a tremendous injustice.

"It's my philosophy that any blessing we receive in this life never comes free as a gift. To own and operate a television station, to be able to produce a film—those blessings come with a tremendous responsibility: When you've finished what you're doing, it has to serve your fellow man in some positive way.

"Doing that feeds something very constructive within me."

Gotta At Least Try

Jump, 62, went hungry for creative sustenance for many years. Born in Dayton, Ohio, he didn't move to California to make a serious stab at acting until he was in his 30s—many years after the bug first bit him.

"From the time I saw my first movie as a kid—some B western—I knew that's what I wanted to do."

His father, Alex, had other ideas. Alex had wanted to be an actor, but didn't make it. He didn't want to see his son head for what he was sure would be disappointment.

But the possibility of failure wasn't as abhorrent to Jump as the thought of ending up behind a desk, not having tried at all. So off he went to…well, not Hollywood. To the University of Kansas, where he majored in speech, thinking it would pave the way to an acting career.

After he graduated, he worked at various jobs at television stations in Kansas and Ohio: writer, production director, and the like. When he was working at a Topeka station, he met the popular leading man Gary Cooper, who was there to tape an interview. "He was being swamped by autograph seekers," recalls Jump. "I looked at him, shrugged my shoulders and said, 'That's the price you pay for fame.' He laughed and his face went down into the next piece of paper.

"After the interview was taped, he came over to me behind the camera and said, 'What are you doing here?' and I said, 'Waiting for a chance to do what you do.' He said, 'You either have to go to New York or California. If you ever decide to come to California, look me up.'

"He died before I ever got a chance to go to California. But in that little moment, he recognized something. With that, and how I felt about my own abilities, I gave it a shot. It was partly his influence that gave me the courage to do it."

Jump packed up his family, moved to California, and knocked on doors. And knocked. And knocked. It started to look as if his father were right. "All the time I was struggling he was saying, 'Come home. Forget that mess, come back here, and get a real job.'" Jump was tempted, but kept doggedly pursuing his dream. "The story of the little engine that could—it's no joke. You keep believing that you can; you keep going until you do it."

He acted in small theaters and after several years got an agent. That agent, through some "embellishments and fabrications," got Jump a part on an episode of *Daniel Boone*.

"If Paul King [the producer of the show] had turned to me, he probably would have found out what a lousy actor I was because I wouldn't have been able to support the lies that my agent was telling."

Through a stroke of luck, the bit part of eight lines turned into eight pages, second billing, and a week's work. "I thought, boy, my career now is really going to be on a roll," Jump recalls. "But the truth is, it was almost a year before I did another job in TV."

Commercials and guest shots trickled in, eventually leading to regular roles on TV, several movies (check out the auctioneer in *Conquest of the Planet of the Apes*), and the role he's best known for: Arthur Carlson on *WKRP in Cincinnati*.

WKRP ran a total of six seasons (1978–82, 1991–92). You can catch the original show in syndication. Look closely and you'll see an American Diabetes Association poster on the wall. The set designers seem to have known what Jump didn't yet.

Ten years ago, Jump was diagnosed with type 2 diabetes. He went on a diet (no more steak-and-kidney pie or Yorkshire pudding) and cranked up his exercise routine (more tennis and golf). He dropped 20 pounds and brought his diabetes under control.

After a few years, he added oral agents to his regimen. Then came the ghosts of Christmas.

Surround With Positive

This past winter, Jump was on the road starring in a version of *A Christmas Carol*. "It was a tough piece to do," he says. "I was onstage for 2½ hours as Scrooge; I had to drive that sucker. And when you come to a local community as the 'star,' everybody's expecting you to perform at an unusually high level, so you have all that emotional stress."

A few creative differences with the director added frustrations. "But you somehow muddle through, and you get a decent review, and the audience jumps on their feet and gives the production a standing ovation. But until that all takes place, there's a great deal of pressure, and that's certainly not a situation in which a diabetic should be working."

Jump's blood glucose levels started creeping up. "Stress is really a troublesome factor when you have diabetes. I also wasn't respecting my diet."

The play finished its run, and Jump went back home in time for the holidays (as relaxing as they always are) and for the January earthquake, which led to a hasty move when his apartment was condemned.

Jump's blood glucose levels hovered in the 200s—sometimes crossing the 300 mark. Finally, he was convinced he needed insulin. "I resisted it," Jump admits. "At first, the doctor said to me, 'I think we should be thinking about insulin.' Later he said, 'I think we should be using insulin.' Then he said to me, 'You don't have a choice anymore. If you want to stay alive and healthy, you're going to have to go on insulin.'

"You think of yourself as a macho sort of guy who can fight off stuff. When you have to start relying on insulin injections, you're no longer your own person. I think that's psychologically one of the factors that kept me from doing it."

He has discovered it isn't so bad after all. "I think I'm going to be very comfortable with this. I wish I had done it a long time ago—I'd probably have saved some nerve damage. Be that as it may, I didn't, and now I'll just have to see how long it takes me to get everything balanced out."

As part of that effort, he's back on a healthy diet. "It's hard to come to grips with the fact that you just can't eat the same things you use to eat. Fortunately I have a wife that watches very closely what I eat and helps me as best she can to stay on the diet."

Jump also works on surrounding himself with the positive—not easy when you have diabetes, he says."Diabetes is probably one of the most insidious, cruel diseases in the book—if you don't take care of it, and you let it get out of control. One of the best ways to keep it under control is with a positive attitude. Yet the disease itself works against this. When that body chemistry gets out of balance, it produces negative feelings: the tiredness, the listlessness, the lack of ambition that become a part of a person with diabetes.

"I have trouble getting out of bed in the morning when my blood sugar has been high. It's very easy to become a couch potato. All of that works directly in favor of the disease.

"You've got to drive yourself to get up and out. When you do, you need to be physical about what you're doing and be smart enough to watch your diet and take your medication. You've got to get out there and press the positive, eliminate the negative, and don't mess with Mr. In-Between. You have to keep talking to yourself; keep telling yourself that you can be the victor.

"Keep a positive attitude, think well-being for yourself, and watch your condition closely. You be the master; don't let it master you."

Do What You Love

To that end, Jump surrounds himself with positives: family and friends, good music (classical, "positive" country-western, light opera), and good books. He walks 3 miles a couple of times a week. "If my schedule were constant, it would be three to four times a week."

Well, his schedule is constant—constantly busy. Jump is still hustling for jobs, just like he did when he first moved to California.

"You go back to the position where you're only as good as your last job. You're still out there knocking on doors. It really doesn't change."

Jump does voice-over work (the people you hear on commercials but never see), and he's going into his sixth year as the Maytag Repairman (look on the lid of Maytag products at the store—that's him). He also does radio, TV, and theater. "I love it all. I'm a glutton," he says.

He'll even do musicals, though it's not his strong suit. He takes voice lessons when he's preparing for a role. "I'm not a singer, so my teacher really has to work with me," he says.

He teaches acting but doesn't encourage his students to take it up as a career. "I tell them: If there's anything else that you can do, don't try to do this business. You must understand the difference between thinking that this is just a nice vocation and being dedicated to a craft. But if you're driven because something inside of you says: 'This is what I'm here to do,' then don't let anyone tell you that you can't."

Jump has three daughters, Cindy, Kiva, and Maggiejo; Cindy and Kiva are actresses. Echoing his own father, Jump tried to dissuade them. "I've done everything in my power, but they want to play the crazy game."

He should know it's useless to try to keep an actor from acting. Jump himself doesn't plan to retire from acting— ever. "If I can remember the lines," he says, "I'll do the part."

Marie McCarren is associate editor of Diabetes Forecast.

Art Shell: Tackling Type 2

by Roger Doughty

This article appeared in *Diabetes Forecast,* January 1996.

During his 15-year career with the Oakland Raiders, left tackle Art Shell never faced an opponent he feared or a fried chicken he didn't like. But that was before he found out he had diabetes.

Shell admits that all those fried chickens, combined with less exercise than he knew he should be getting, did what some of the meanest, nastiest guys in the National Football League could never do—put him out of commission and into the hospital.

Shell's hospital stint, which he calls "the episode," occurred during training camp prior to the 1993 season, when he was head coach of the Raiders. It lasted less than 24 hours, but his brief hospitalization was chow for the newshounds—the story was picked up by hundreds of newspapers around the country. Never has anyone been diagnosed with type 2 diabetes with more fanfare. But the big media splash upset him.

"I knew what was going to happen," says Shell, who is now an offensive line coach with the Kansas City Chiefs. "It scared a lot of my friends. All they heard was, 'Art's in the hospital.' They thought, 'My God, what's going on?'"

What was going on was pretty unusual. Although millions of Americans have been diagnosed with type 2, the "silent" diabetes, few get sent off to the hospital on the spot and fewer still have reporters clamoring to get all the details.

Of the estimated 16 million Americans who have diabetes, slightly more than 95 percent are thought to have type 2. There may be no symptoms, yet a person's blood glucose levels can be high or erratic for years prior to diagnosis—all the time doing damage to kidneys, blood vessels, and nerves.

"I felt fine," says Shell. "The only thing that was going on was that I was urinating quite frequently. I hated to leave camp, but my numbers were up there around 700 [mg/dl] and the doctor said, 'I don't know how you're walking around—you should be passed out. You need to be in the hospital.' He was right. It was the best thing to do."

During his brief convalescence, Shell's health care team took away the play book he relied on to run the Raiders and sat him down in front of a TV screen. "I had seven videos about diabetes I had to watch, and I learned a lot," he says enthusiastically. "I found there's no one age group affected by diabetes. They had 9-year-old kids with the problem. Anybody can have diabetes."

In addition to using the downtime to increase his knowledge of diabetes, Shell took insulin shots to lower his blood sugar, then was switched to oral medication. "The doctor waived me off that when I got to the point where I didn't need it anymore," the coach recalls. "I don't take any medication now, but I do keep an eye on those numbers."

A Hard Guy to Hurt

You can't blame Shell for being concerned about what his friends and fans would think when they found out he was in the hospital. During his decade and a half as one of the greatest offensive left tackles in the history of professional football, Shell matched brains and brawn against the best in the business on 207 occasions (the third highest total in Raider history). That included one stretch of 156 games in a row, a rare accomplishment in an occupation in which broken bones, pulled muscles, and painful sprains routinely sideline even the most well-conditioned athletes. He rarely came away with an injury he considered to be anything more than an occupational hazard.

In the course of a typical work day, Shell was called upon to continually smash his well-muscled, 6-foot-5-inch, 285-pound body into opposing players intent on decapitating Raider quarterbacks. That's what left tackles do.

Because most quarterbacks are right-handed, their heads and bodies are turned to the right as they set up to pass or hand off to a running back. Without the benefit of rearview mirrors on their helmets, they can't see what's coming from the left. To take advantage of this situation, opposing teams usually put their best pass rusher on the right side of the line, giving him a clear shot at the blind side of the signal caller. Only one man stands between the pass rusher and the fame and fortune that come to those who consistently clobber the quarterback—none other than the left tackle.

The tackles usually triumph in their classic confrontations with would-be decapitators, so the TV cameras turn elsewhere to find something more exciting to show us. On the rare occasions when they fail, we are subjected to outlandish displays of ostentatious celebration by the victorious intruders. Nothing annoys a left tackle more than such unrestrained behavior.

As many a pass rusher has learned the hard way, it can be downright dangerous to antagonize a tackle by engaging in excessive high jinks after a successful sack. Tackles have an opportunity to exact revenge when their team runs the ball. On those occasions, they try to annihilate anyone attempting to impede the ball carrier's path to the end zone. The great gusto and cruel precision with which ticked-off tackles proceed to carry out these assignments has caused many a defensive end to adopt a more docile demeanor.

A Thankless Task

For a long time, most football fans didn't know, or seem to care, what left tackles did. John Madden, who coached Shell before leaving the Raiders and ascending to the broadcasting booth, has often lavished praise on these men who combine unusual size with unusual speed, but his has long been a voice in the wilderness. Then *Sports Illustrated* (*SI*) hit the stands in September 1994 with a pro football preview issue complete with a cover story extolling the exploits of the mighty men who take such a pounding protecting the passers.

According to *SI*, prerequisites for successful left tackles include strength, quickness, nimble feet, long arms, and plenty of stamina. "In short," declared the author, "you want a gigantic Baryshnikov." So how did Shell measure up to these standards? "Better than anyone else, ever," the magazine concluded in a separate story devoted to his illustrious career.

Few challenge *SI*'s assertion that Shell was the greatest left tackle ever, but there's no scientific way it can be documented. The greatness of quarterbacks, running backs, or receivers is relatively easy to measure in terms of passes completed, touchdowns scored, or yardage gained. Pass rushers are rated by sacks, hurries, and fumbles forced or recovered. But a left tackle's finest moments come when nothing happens—when he nullifies the efforts of his opponent. No statistics are kept regarding nullification, but Shell's peers, the men who played with and against him, argue that when it came to making nothing happen, Art Shell was unsurpassed.

Shell retired from the game with two Super Bowl rings on his powerful fingers, leaving behind a host of battered opponents who were delighted when he hung up his helmet and became a Raider assistant coach in 1983. In 1989, the year he was elected to the Hall of Fame, the Raiders named him head coach, making Shell the first black American to hold that post in NFL history. He remained with the Raiders through the 1994 season, compiling a record of 54–38, guiding the team to three playoff appearances, and winning Coach of the Year honors in 1990.

Since joining the Kansas City Chiefs for the '95 season, Shell's winning ways have continued. At press time, the Chiefs were 11–2, and had clinched the AFC-West title.

Diabetes Breaks Through

Diabetes snuck up on Shell. It had to, because unlike the typical American male who would rather swim naked through shark-infested waters than have a physical, Shell has had so many physicals that he gives having another about as much thought as you and I might to brushing our teeth.

"You get a print-out so you can see everything," Shell says, describing the diagnostic feedback provided by today's hi-tech pro football physicals, "but nothing ever showed up." Still, he wasn't totally surprised the day his glucose reading went off the charts. "My dad had diabetes, so I was aware that at some point, if I didn't watch myself, I could get it."

So was Shell "watching himself" in the summer of '93? No way. Ten years of coaching in the pressure-packed environment of the NFL, where winning is everything, combined with frequent travel, too many meals on the run, and a lack of exercise finally caught up with the man most football fans considered invincible.

"I was foolish," Shell acknowledges. "When you're coaching, you get away from doing exercise. You get your mind bogged down on so many things that you don't do it. And you don't always eat properly. The night before the episode, I had some fried chicken, and it all just boiled over."

Art's Winning Ways

Shell won't say how much weight he gained during that decade between his last hurrah as a player and the arrival of "the episode"—or how much he's shed since—but he's willing to tell you how he did it and share his four-point training program with anyone who will listen. The nice thing about this routine is that you don't have to be a Hall of Fame athlete to do it. All you have to do is be like Art—smart.

■ You are what you eat.
"I don't eat like I used to," Coach Shell admits. At home his wife, Janice, runs interference in the diet department, but on the road, he's on his own. "You just have to order the proper stuff," the coach says. "I used to eat all the fried foods. Now I eat a turkey sandwich with lettuce and tomato, and I don't put anything on it. Moderation is the key. Once you learn how to eat, you find out it isn't too bad."

■ Walk, don't run.
"I swore I would never run when I got through playing," says the man who logged many a mile on the football field,

"but I didn't say I wouldn't walk. You can get just as much out of walking as you can out of jogging, and you won't hurt your bones or muscles. I walk 2 miles a day and get it down to 25 or 26 minutes in a fast-paced walk. When you get a nice brisk walk going every day, you'll find that your pace will pick up. You'll go faster and faster. And if you don't walk one day, you'll feel bad."

■ Kick back and relax.
Coaching in the NFL is very near the top of the list when it comes to high-pressure jobs. So what does a guy like Art Shell do to relax? "If I'm with a group, I like to play cards," the coach says with a smile. "If I'm by myself, I like to watch historical movies, especially war movies, because I associate the battlefield strategies with the game plan. I love watching Patton just to see how he'd say, 'We're going to swing over here, then we're going to swing over there, then we're going to hit 'em right in the mouth.' I like that kind of stuff."

■ Get the word out.
"I've talked to my sons (Art III and Christopher) and I've talked to my three younger brothers and I tell them, 'You guys have to beware now. Diabetes runs in our family, so you have to be ready for it.' So far they've been getting their physicals and having their checkups and watching what they eat."

Whether he's speaking to family members or to folks he doesn't know who might be at risk for diabetes, Coach Shell's message is the same: Take care of yourself. Although his main interest in life is getting positive results from teams with no more than 11 players, if he has to be on a squad with almost 16 million other people, he wants them to be winners too.

Roger Doughty is a freelance writer and avid football fan living in Minneapolis, Minnesota.

Hats Off to Michelle McGann

by *Marcia Levine Mazur*

This article appeared in *Diabetes Forecast,* April 1995.

Michelle McGann, signature hat planted firmly on her head, steps up to the tee, tests the wind, and smokes the ball a whopping 260 yards.

Her fans gasp, shake their heads in disbelief, then burst into applause. They've just witnessed one of the longest drives in women's golf today.

The 25-year-old McGann has been thrilling them on the women's pro golf circuit for 6 years now. No wonder. She's got finesse as well as power, finishing among the top 10—often among the top 5—in numerous Ladies Professional Golf Association (LPGA) tournaments. She also led the LPGA Tour in driving distance in 1992 with an average drive of 252.1 yards.

"Michelle has it all," says Australian Jan Stephenson, one of the all-time top 10 LPGA money winners, and one of the first women to bring glamour onto the green. She counts herself among McGann's admirers. Stephenson adds, "Michelle is attractive, has a great personality, and most important, she can really play. In fact, Michelle is the newcomer with the most potential."

McGann is no slouch when it comes to commercial endorsements either; she is possibly the most sought-after player in the LPGA. At a statuesque 5 feet 11 inches, McGann has looks and presence as well as talent.

However, although she's already banked nearly 1 million dollars in earnings, she has yet to win an LPGA tournament.

Surprise

That may surprise the nongolfer, but it's not news to those familiar with the game. "There are girls here who have played for 20 years and not won a tournament yet," McGann explains. "Some play to win, but some just want to make a living."

McGann is one woman who definitely wants to win.

Yet when McGann was 13 in her home town of West Palm Beach, Florida, she was afraid she'd never play golf. Like any 13-year-old, she didn't understand what it meant to be diagnosed with something called type 1 diabetes.

"My mom is a nurse," McGann explains. "When she saw all the water I was drinking and the weight I'd lost, she took me to her office and tested me for diabetes." Although no one else in the family has the disease, Bernadette McGann had guessed correctly. Her daughter did, indeed, have diabetes.

"I wondered if I could still lead a normal life," McGann recalls, "or keep on with my plans. It had been my long-term goal to be a pro golfer."

Not the usual dream of a 13-year-old, but McGann had fallen in love with golf the first time she popped a ball onto the fairway. That happened when she was 8.

"It started by accident. My dad played often and I went with him one day just for something to do. I loved it. I began spending entire days on the course. Since it was owned by a patient of my mom's, I felt comfortable there even though I was so young."

She continued playing golf almost daily. And 5 years later, when she was diagnosed with diabetes, she fought her concerns about the disease, and determined that it would not break up her love affair with golf. "In fact, I knew almost as soon as I got back to the course that my diabetes wasn't going to handicap me," she says.

Rough Spots

Diabetes does sometimes throw her life into the rough, however. "I have ups and downs, of course. At times the adrenalin is really flowing, and it's hard to know how much insulin to take. Other times I know something is wrong because I feel tired and my swing gets weaker. But when you're a professional you have to keep going."

Jan Stephenson adds, "I think the most important thing about her diabetes is that she doesn't use it as an excuse although it would be easy."

McGann did have a serious insulin reaction during a junior tournament in Illinois. "Back then, junior players weren't allowed to talk to anyone during a tournament. We even carried our own bags, so I couldn't tell my parents how I was feeling, and I passed out on the fairway. Fortunately it's a lot different now," she adds.

Her parents were at her side in a minute, of course. But Bucky and Bernadette McGann never stopped supporting their daughter's desire to stay with the game. Never mind the energy-draining tournaments, each stretching 3 to 4 weeks in a row, from January through September, and sometimes beyond. Never mind the endless days of practice before, during, and after the tournaments, often under a brutal sun.

And never mind that she has diabetes. McGann works hard to keep her blood glucose in control, staying in close touch with her endocrinologist, testing twice a day, and taking two insulin injections a day. "But I never inject on the golf course," she adds.

She carries a quick sugar source in case of an insulin reaction, as well as fruit, crackers, and often a peanut butter sandwich in her golf bag. "You're out there for 5 hours, and you can't stop for lunch during a tournament," she says.

Michelle often plays with Sherri Turner, another member of the LPGA who travels the pro Tour while managing her own type 1 diabetes. (*Diabetes Forecast,* "Lady With A Drive," August 1989, pp. 28–31.)

Caddy Dad

The McGanns encourage Michelle to stick with her career. They feel that all that exercise is actually a bonus, helping her control her diabetes.

Bucky McGann even left his own lawn maintenance business to travel the LPGA Tour and caddy for his daughter. "It's very lonely out there," Michelle explains. "And a good caddy, someone you are comfortable with, is difficult to find. My dad knows my swing and things like that. It works out great."

Her 16-year-old brother, J.C., sometimes caddies too. ("We watch him for any sign of diabetes. So far there are none," McGann adds.)

From High School To LPGA

The McGann family also respected Michelle's decision to leapfrog over college and go directly into professional golf. "I could have gotten a golf scholarship to just about any school I wanted, the University of Miami, Duke, Stanford, UCLA," she says.

But, although McGann was a good student, she didn't feel comfortable spending another 4 years in classes. "I knew pro golf was what I wanted and I knew it would be stressful, but so would college," she explains. "And with golf there would be all that exercise."

She had already been three-time Florida State Junior Champion, and that in a state that reveres its golf. In 1987 she was ranked top junior golfer by *Golf Magazine* and *Golf Digest*. She won the U.S. Golf Association's Junior Girls Championship that same year.

But it was her impressive showing in the U.S. Open in 1988—she entered as an amateur—that convinced her she could compete with the best. She qualified for the LPGA in 1989, when she was only 18 years old, a rare occurrence.

Has she ever regretted choosing pro golf over college? "Never," she says. "I did the right thing."

The Fad Hatter

The trademark hats came along a few years later, in 1991. Although she has signed a commercial endorsement with a clothing designer and several food companies— including one that markets sugar-free products—and is considering offers from sports equipment manufacturers, it's her fashion statements that take the limelight.

She knows the crowds look for the red lipstick, wide belt, necklace, dangling earrings, and coordinated color scheme when she steps onto the course. "People would wonder what was wrong if I didn't dress up to play," McGann says, laughing.

But it's the saucy wide-brimmed hats that really have them talking. And that started the way it might with any fashion-conscious woman.

"I had played well one week and made $35,000. I've always loved dressing well, and I went on a shopping spree. I saw these cute hats and decided to wear one at the U.S. Women's Open in Fort Worth. I got very positive comments, so I wore them all the time. People began recognizing me by my hats."

About a year later, a California hat company, which knew a good thing when it saw it, signed her on as a sponsor and, voila! instead of buying her own hats, she now earns income wearing theirs.

Although the hats are marketed, the ones she wears are specially styled to match her outfits.

Later this year, women will also be able to snap on a Michelle McGann charm bracelet or earrings from a whole line of Michelle McGann jewelry. "The jewelry has been designed by a different company, but they'll coordinate it with the hats. Kind of sun-fun fashion," McGann says.

All this means that Michelle McGann doesn't travel light. But her proud dad often does double-duty making sure her bags and boxes make it to the next tournament.

Michelle is particularly pleased that women golfers can now display their femininity on the golf course. "All of this would never have been possible a couple of generations back. But what's wrong with looking good while you're playing?" she asks. "We're women. We should look like women."

Waiting To Win

Although McGann gets innumerable calls, letters, and faxes from men who'd like to meet her, she's not interested. "My focus right now is golf. That's what I'm concentrating on," she says.

"I've learned a lot these past years, and I keep improving. I know the wins will come. Players who win early don't necessarily stay on top," she adds.

"Sometimes it just takes a few breaks, but when I get my first win, it will be easy, and the next will be even easier.

"Besides, I'm having lots of fun."

Marcia Levine Mazur is senior editor of Diabetes Forecast.

Fran Carpentier: On Parade

by Marcia Levine Mazur

This article appeared in *Diabetes Forecast,* May 1995.

"**T**hey promised me glamour. They lied." Fran Carpentier, a senior editor of *Parade,* America's largest weekly magazine, whips out words quicker than a New York minute.

"Here I am, sitting behind my desk, wearing running shoes, eating a turkey on whole wheat, and wiping my brow with a Kleenex. What ever happened to expense account lunches at the Four Seasons?"

The words tumble out like a Joan Rivers monologue. "Been here 15 years—my God, it's really long!—juggling ten balls at a time, running from meeting to deadline to the next crisis. We're a weekly, so there's no downtime. And you know what? I love it."

Carpentier is fast and funny, and passionate about her disease. "Diabetes? Sure I have diabetes. Had it 26 years. And I'm the world's greatest diabetic. Whatever the doctor tells me to do, I do. It's true. It's true. I even know all my exchanges by heart. Ask me. Go ahead. Ask me."

Age

"How old am I?" she repeats, then admonishes herself in a stage whisper, "Have some self-respect, Fran. Lie. Lie." Instead she laughs and blurts out, "All right, so I'm 40, which means that, back when I was diagnosed, diabetes treatment was akin to witchcraft."

Stories pour out. "The doctors...God love 'em...they sent your blood sample to the lab and a day or so later a reading came back. And what did the reading mean? No one knew.

"I used to call the doctor after my urine test—no blood glucose readings then—and report, 'Doctor, my sugar is high.' He'd say, 'Fran, run coverage.' I'd say, 'Run coverage? Doctor, are we making this up as we go along?'"

Then she'd inject anywhere from 5 to 7 units of insulin. "My God! Today we know that casually taking an extra 5 units of insulin can lower your blood sugar to smithereens. "Remember, 25 years ago we diabetics had no idea what our blood sugars were. We'd be walking around with a blood glucose level of 250 [mg/dl] every day and not know it.

"Back then, having diabetes was like crossing the ocean in a raft when you didn't know how to swim. And neither did your doctor. They just didn't know."

Teen Tribulations

Although Carpentier was diagnosed with type 1 diabetes as a 14-year-old in Brooklyn, N.Y., she still remembers the I-feel-like-I'm-going-to-die weakness, the hunger, the parched mouth. "I was so dry I had stopped salivating," she says.

They tested her urine with a test strip, the only way to check for diabetes in 1969. "When they found out I was diabetic, my mother became hysterical and fainted.

"When they told me I'd be injecting myself with a needle every day, I said, 'What? Are you kidding?'"

Members of her Italian family came from miles around to mourn her. "Fran has diabetes," they said. "Fran is dying." Her mother and aunts told her never even to dream of having a baby. "I thought they must be right. What did I know?"

Diabetes was an especially frightening diagnosis for an adolescent. "Kids can be so cruel," Carpentier adds. "I had two best friends. One said, 'Fran, are you going to die?' The other said, 'Is diabetes contagious?' I said, 'Yes. And I'm going to breathe all over you.'

"On the other hand, pity is not such a bad thing," Carpentier adds, laughing. "You get attention, a little TLC. I could live with pity. Well, for a little while."

Read, Learn, Obey

The 14-year-old plunged into her subject, learned all she could about diabetes, and reassured her family that she wasn't going to die—and that she could have a baby.

"I became every doctor's dream patient. Still am," she says. "I tell myself, 'The doctor is the Commandant of Blood Sugar Control'; and I bow and say, 'I obey. I obey.' But of course I wouldn't do that if I didn't have complete trust in my doctor."

Carpentier's words slow to a gallop. "But listen, this is the best time in the world to have diabetes. It's true. It's true. We have low-fat foods, self-monitoring, different insulins. Imagine! You can tailor your regimen to your lifestyle.

"But there's a downside—or maybe it's an upside. Responsibility for our health is thrown back at us. We folks with diabetes are the masters of our fate now. And, trust me, this is not a disease for the cranky. Spoiled brats need not apply."

The pace picks up. "Listen, what you have here is one major pain-in-the-neck disease, and probably the most frustrating. Every now and then I can't maintain control no matter what I do. It's disheartening. Even though you are doing everything right—taking your insulin at the right time, following your meal plan, all that—you still can't get the numbers you want."

Carpentier has had no hint of complications after 26 years of careful control. Diabetes certainly didn't stop her from graduating Phi Beta Kappa with a journalism degree from New York University, or interfere with her becoming editor-in-chief of *Lady's Circle* magazine at 24. "Ye Gods, was I ever 24?" she says.

According to Carpentier, being hired by *Parade* was one of the greatest pluses of her life. "I love it here. Every day is stimulating, challenging. And I can say these people are the best in the business."

The other great pluses in her life were marrying Dr. Ira Salom, an internist and geriatrician with LaGuardia and Mount Sinai Hospitals, and giving birth to Benjamin Francis almost a year ago, all while keeping her diabetes in near-perfect control.

Enough Already

Still, she's had enough of diabetes.

"I need a new disease, something less labor intensive, something sexy," she says. "About 10 years ago a slew of Hollywood starlets got hypoglycemia (low blood glucose). It was mysterious, exotic. And the best part, only skinny nymphets got it.

"But diabetes? That's another image. It's like that old *The Andy Griffith Show*. It wouldn't have surprised anyone if Opie came home one day and said, 'Guess what, Pa? Aunt Bee got diabetes.'"

A deep breath. "Another thing. I hate it when people say, 'If you have high blood sugars it must be because you're stressed,' and I think, 'Oh, please. I wouldn't be stressed if I didn't have high blood sugars.'"

She doesn't care for the "You don't look like you have diabetes" observation either. "Hello. What does diabetes look like? Do I have to be gray and pallid to have diabetes?"

Nothing gray or pallid about Fran Carpentier. The fit 5 foot ½ inch—"Don't forget the half"—120 pounder has returned to her pre-pregnancy weight. "I thought I was going to turn into Roseanne Barr after the birth," she says, "but when I was pregnant you could never catch me eating anything I shouldn't. After all, it was for the baby."

No More Whispers

The 1990s have brought Carpentier new pride in her disease. "I used to whisper to the waiter, 'Fish, broiled, no sauce. Salad, no dressing.' Now I shout it. Now people look at me with respect. Respect, I tell you! Everyone is health conscious—it's trendy. But, hey, we diabetics were here first."

She thanks science, too. "All the advances, the DCCT, the technology. So many breakthroughs—genes causing diabetes. Finally, we're on the map.

"Oh, and the pump. Wait. Let me tell you about my insulin pump."

The Big Beep

"First, I had to get used to having catheters hanging out of my clothes. Then, a few months later, I started beeping.

I had an important appointment and I began beeping, beeping, beeping. I called up the pump company. 'I'm beeping!' I told them."

They asked where her new batteries were. "Batteries? You mean I'm supposed to carry batteries too? I had to run to three stores—beeping—and find the right batteries."

She has good words about the pump, though.

"Nothing made me confront my diabetes as much as wearing an insulin pump. With the pump you are on [fast-acting], Regular insulin. If there is any interruption—a tiny air bubble in the catheter—you could go hours without getting your insulin. And you wouldn't know it.

"So you have to be extremely vigilant about blood testing. A pump is not for the faint of heart, believe me. We pumpers are the Olympians of diabetics."

Her husband adds, "And you know where she keeps her pump? In a black elastic leather garter on her upper thigh. It has a little pouch for cigarettes and the pump just fits there.

"It started when we went to Italy after we were married and I bought Fran some beautiful fitted dresses. She needed somewhere to wear the pump so it wouldn't show under the dresses. First we went to a police supply store in New York and bought a holster for a concealed weapon. But a few months later we hit pay dirt in Greenwich Village. We happened upon the garter."

Carpentier sums up the find: "The garter has changed my life. We who wear the pump have to be resourceful. Yes. Believe me. It's true. It's true."

Shakespeare?

Ira and Fran are so in love, friends think of them as the Romeo and Juliet of Third Avenue. ("But," Carpentier says, "we look like the Mertzes. You know, Lucy and Ricky's neighbors.") Unlike the Mertzes, however, they are ecstatic when they talk about each other.

"We each had been married before, and each had a bad time of it," Carpentier says, recalling those post-divorce days. "I knew there would be a light at the end of the tunnel, but it was such a long tunnel, and every unmarried career woman has been in it. Oh, the horrors of dating. Don't ask."

Theirs is a New York romance: The Saloms found each other at a meeting of the Board of Directors of the alumni association of New York University.

"Right away I knew she had everything, smarts—she's a Phi Beta Kappa—heart—the personality of Mother Teresa—and great gams," Salom says of his wife.

Carpentier adds in soft tones, "I adore my husband. Oh, I love him so much. We're so happy. We have a baby now, and you know my greatest fear?" She whispers, "That I'm asking for too much."

What Am I Doing Here?

The family lives in a Manhattan apartment many blocks from the *Parade* offices, and Carpentier takes the bus there every day. She resumed work 4 months after Benjamin was born.

"We have a marvelous babysitter. I love my work, and I get a lot out of it. I also believe it's important to be a happy mom.

"But sometimes I think, 'I worked so hard to have this baby. What am I doing at the office?'"

Love My Diet

Carpentier is optimistic, always looking for the positives, especially about her diabetes. "For instance," she says, "I love my food. I truly mean it. They call it a restricted diet, but I say, 'No way.' When I travel and have a problem getting the fresh fruits and vegetables I eat, I'm miserable."

She adds, "You can't believe how carefully I do what I'm told. I test my blood four to six times a day, follow all the other rigors of tight control, and it's paid off. I am in wonderful health."

"Fran is a great patient," her husband adds. "I wish I had patients like Fran."

"Why not?" Carpentier adds. "But I have this recurring nightmare. What if they cure me? How would I spend my snack time? What would I look forward to?

"Never mind. Go ahead and cure me. I'll think of something."

Marcia Levine Mazur is senior editor of Diabetes Forecast.

Bill Clotworthy: Master of Change

by Marcia Levine Mazur

This article appeared in *Diabetes Forecast,* April 1996.

At age 65, Bill Clotworthy had a zinger of a career change. He chucked 12 years as censor for *TV's Saturday Night Live* (yes, they have one), and another 30 years as program supervisor and producer of TV commercials, and became—hold your hat—a presidential historian.

And no one is more surprised than he.

"I left *Saturday Night Live* because it just seemed time to go," he explains. "And I got into presidential history because I tried to sell a free-lance article about insults presidential candidates have hurled at each other since Washington's day." The article died, but the idea of a book on presidential residences and libraries took root. Clotworthy offered it to several publishers, and a small Florida firm took him up on it.

The result: *Homes and Libraries of the Presidents* is now in book stores, *A Visitors' Guide To Presidential Sites* is due out this summer, and a third title is in the works.

Ask Bill Clotworthy about his books, and he'll gladly discuss them. Ask about the diet-and-exercise regimen that helps him control type 2 diabetes, and he'll be delighted to explain it. But ask for information about his career in TV, and his face will light up and he'll offer you a chair. "Those were great days," he'll begin. "And I loved every minute of them—right from the start."

The Golden Age

It all started in 1948. Clotworthy was 22 years old, fresh out of the Navy and Syracuse University, and away from his home town of Westfield, N.J.

He'd been hired as a page at NBC, where an accident of timing put him backstage for the TV debuts of Sid Caesar, Milton Berle, Perry Como, and even Howdy Doody.

NBC also put him to work in one of the industry's most celebrated television studios, 8H.

"It was converted from radio and it may be the most acoustically perfect studio ever built," he recalls, "because NBC built it for one of the most prestigious radio shows ever put on the air, *Arturo Toscanini and the NBC Symphony Orchestra.*" (Clotworthy didn't know it then, but he and studio 8H would meet again.)

Although he enjoyed life as a page, Clotworthy wanted more than a page's view of show biz. So he went after a job with BBD&O, the fabled New York ad agency, and landed it.

That job put Clotworthy in the heart of the newborn television industry; back then advertisers and their agencies, not networks, owned and produced most TV shows.

A Short 20 Years

BBD&O transferred Clotworthy to Hollywood for "a short stint" that turned into a 20-year assignment.

"It was in the early '50s," Clotworthy recalls. "If you weren't around then, let me tell you about it. Those were the days when you wrangled an invitation to the neighbors, even if you couldn't stand them, just because they had a television set.

"And you caught shows such as *Your Hit Parade* with Snooky Lanson, Eileen Wilson, and Dorothy Collins." (Remember the Lucky Strike bullseye?) You watched a young band leader named Horace Heidt, and never missed an episode of *Dragnet* with Jack Webb. Naturally, you laughed your head off at *You Bet Your Life* with Groucho Marx.

Then there were Jack Benny, Danny Kaye, George Burns and Gracie Allen, and Bing Crosby.

Clotworthy worked with all these stars and others back when TV was a "live" medium.

"When I first went to Hollywood many of the advertisers—our clients—owned their TV programs. And I was their representative on the set.

"My work ranged from the serious—writing and producing Ronald Reagan's host material for *General Electric Theater*, for example—to the absurd—checking the set to make sure there were no gas ranges there.

"I supervised production and directed hundreds of commercials. My work meant I got to know all the personalities on the show," he explains.

On occasion the stars surprised him. "One Christmas we asked Bing Crosby to read a public service announcement. Instead of reading directly from the page, he glanced at the script, set it aside, and did the whole thing perfectly from memory. I had always known Crosby was a quiet, pleasant man, but until then I hadn't realized how bright he was."

Dropping The Curtain

What's it like working on live TV? "There's a kind of bedlam backstage just before the show goes on. The clock is ticking and people are rehearsing, screaming for rewrites, trying on costumes. After all, there was no second chance to get it right.

"It was exciting for everyone. But," Clotworthy adds, "celebrity can be a terrible burden. There's such a lack of privacy. I found that most stars put up a protective shield offstage. Even Groucho wasn't always funny away from the set."

Never Enough

Clotworthy's relationship with most of the actors was strictly professional, but he knew one well enough to call him Ronnie.

His friend's full name is Ronald Reagan, host of the *General Electric Theater*. Clotworthy smiles remembering how close Ron and Nancy were even then.

"When we'd get to the set, he'd call Nancy, say he'd be home soon, and tell her he loved her. When we'd finished, he'd call again, say he was on his way home, and tell her he loved her."

When Clotworthy suggested that might be a bit much, Reagan told him, "You can't say it enough."

Although Clotworthy didn't take Reagan's advice about phone messages, he had an idyllic homelife. He married Joyce Holland in 1954, and the couple had three children.

But the good times didn't last.

Joyce became seriously ill. In 1963 she underwent open heart surgery, which was still a relatively rudimentary procedure in those days. She didn't make it.

Clotworthy was left to raise three children (two boys, one girl), all under the age of eight.

He managed, and 3 years later, he met and married Angela Bailey, a widow with four children. "We had seven children between us, and then one more together. There was a time when we had seven teenagers under one roof. It was madness."

Back To New York

After 20 years of working in Hollywood, BBD&O suddenly recalled Clotworthy to New York. He, Angela, and the four youngest children trekked across the country to the East Coast.

"I was in my 50s then, and probably going through a mid-life crisis," Clotworthy recalls, "but I just wasn't happy in my new job at BBD&O."

When a friend told him about an opening at NBC, he applied.

The Incredible "No" Man

The position was listed as Director of Program Standards, but its real title was "censor." Clotworthy got the job.

Technically, he was responsible for a number of programs, including *The Cosby Show* and *Late Night With David Letterman*. But they needed little attention.

The job's real challenge came from a group of talented young people who were stretching the limits of good taste and giving studio execs the jitters. The show was called *Saturday Night Live* (*SNL*).

"I'd never even seen it," Clotworthy recalls. But in 1979, he was signed on as moral guardian of the up-and-coming show.

For the next 12 years it was Bill Clotworthy who decided whether skits about anything from mastectomies to pedophilia, animal rights to alcoholism, made it into American homes.

"It wasn't just blue-lining dirty words," he explains. "I had to decide things like how much pubic hair can be shown on a statue, and how much of a rear end could be exposed during a proctology sketch. Of course, the main problems dealt with sex, drugs, violence, and racial and ethnic stereotyping.

"And if you think the things that got onto *Saturday Night Live* skirted the edge of acceptability, you should have seen what we didn't allow on the air!" he adds.

Although Clotworthy arrived after the show's premier and some time after John Belushi and Dan Aykroyd had left, he worked with most of the now-famous cast members including Jim Belushi, Bill Murray, Billy Crystal, Jane Curtin, Eddie Murphy, and Gilda Radner.

"Gilda was the world's sweetheart," he recalls. "Everybody adored her, and I remember the day she passed away. It was a Saturday morning, a show day, and you could cut the gloom backstage with a knife. That was the most difficult show we ever did. Talk about 'the show must go on.'"

Deja Vu

For Bill Clotworthy there was a *deja vu* quality about *SNL*. "By the time I came back to New York, it was probably the only live television show still on the air."

And wonder of wonders, he was back in studio 8H again. "There I was, some 27 years after I started, back in live TV and back in the same studio. The place is still going strong, too. In fact, I think NBC will probably use it again to broadcast election results this November."

Angela wasn't thrilled with her husband's long hours—especially Wednesday through Saturday, when tensions on the set wound tighter and tighter, and he was sometimes needed there until after midnight.

Otherwise, the new life the family had was pretty good.

Then history seemed to repeat itself. Angela became ill with breast cancer, and she, too, passed away after a long illness.

"I do not recommend widowhood for anyone," Clotworthy says. "You plan to retire with someone. You think you are going to do all kinds of wonderful things together and then that other person passes away and there you are, by yourself, your wonderful plans dashed against the wall."

Fortunately, Clotworthy has always been a great believer in keeping busy. He went on working after Angela died, and he went on caring for himself, taking a medical exam annually.

Yet Another Change

Six years ago he heard something at that exam that knocked him on his heels. His doctor announced that Bill had type 2 diabetes.

The diagnosis was a stunner because Clotworthy felt fine, had no symptoms, and was no more than 6 or 7 pounds overweight.

"Talk about a silent disease," he adds.

The doctor put his patient on medication, but Clotworthy had a bad reaction to it, and decided to attempt to control his disease with diet and exercise.

"I had given up smoking years ago and I figured if I could do that, I could do anything."

First he dispensed with fried foods and the occasional alcoholic drink he'd enjoyed. Then he began reserving ice cream for special occasions.

Clotworthy also started walking 30 minutes a day every day, or running up and down stairs if the weather was bad.

He also became a member of a committee that redesigned the image of the American Diabetes Association. "I don't recall the details," he says. "I know it was a group effort, but we came up with the slogan: Until there's a cure, there's the American Diabetes Association."

Discipline, Discipline

Although Clotworthy admits that sometimes he slips, he has been controlling his diabetes through diet and exercise for 6 years. "The key," he says, "is discipline."

"I take my blood glucose readings regularly, go in every 6 months for a glycohemoglobin, see an eye doctor regularly, and stay in touch with my dietitian."

Clotworthy lives with his daughter, Lynn, but cooks for himself. "I never used to eat veggies, but now I eat them every day, beans and stuff like that. And even though I eat alone, I eat a balanced diet with healthy foods. I don't even buy frozen dinners. I grill and broil or bake everything.

"And I have got to tell you that *Forecast* helps. It reminds me that, hey, I may feel great, but I have to keep taking care of myself.

"It's particularly tough when you have a disease with no clear symptoms, nothing that says you're sick. You have to keep reminding yourself that you have diabetes, that it's real."

He adds, "My brother's 4-year-old granddaughter, Samantha, was recently diagnosed with type 1 diabetes. She takes four insulin shots a day and I tell myself that if she can do that, I can certainly do without a piece of cake."

Clotworthy still believes in keeping busy, and he travels the country researching his presidential books. He also speaks about them or about his show biz days to interested groups. "I enjoy life," he adds, "but make no mistake, life and diabetes are more difficult when you're by yourself."

But on his own or not, Bill Clotworthy has rung up the curtain on yet another career, writing books about the presidents. And today he has as much enthusiasm for the pronouncements of George Washington and Thomas Jefferson as he ever had for the antics of Jack Benny and Groucho Marx.

Marcia Levine Mazur is senior editor of Diabetes Forecast.

Dizzy Gillespie: Blowing Strong

by Marcia Levine Mazur

This interview was conducted when Dizzy Gillespie was 70 years old and appeared in *Diabetes Forecast*, September 1988.

His name was "Dizzy," but Mrs. Gillespie's son was nobody's fool. Dizzy Gillespie was one of the most renowned jazzmen of the 20th century, a virtuoso trumpeter, composer, innovator, band leader, and international ambassador for more than 50 years. And he didn't stop living his life on fast-forward right up until the end of it.

Dizzy—a name he got from his onstage antics—puffed out his cheeks and blew his bent-bell trumpet from Copenhagen to Cairo, Jerusalem to Ankara, Nairobi to Rio. And all across the United States. He performed solo or with a quartet, quintet, or big band at least 200 times a year, even in his 70s.

At age 68, he was handed "one of the biggest surprises of my life." That was when Dizzy learned he had type 2 diabetes. The disease was no stranger. One brother had diabetes, and two sisters died of its complications.

Dizzy carried another vivid memory. He talked of Mrs. Amanda Harrington, a childhood neighbor he called "almost a second mother. She taught me how to say my alphabet. The first trumpet I played on was her son James's.

"She had diabetes. One day a sore toe developed into gangrene. That was in the early '20s. She had to have her leg cut off. I still get cold chills when I think about it," he said.

Sweetmouth Fool

That may be one reason Dizzy acted fast after his own diagnosis. "I was a fat man then, nearly 220 pounds. I'm about 5 foot 10½. The doctor told me, 'You better lose weight.' He scared me so much I think I lost weight by the time I got home."

Diabetes changed Dizzy's approach to food. "I was a sweetmouth fool," he said. "Now I don't put any sugar in my body. I don't use sugar in my coffee, not even artificial. My major diet is fish and chicken—no red meat." Also, Dizzy's Baha'i religion did not allow alcohol.

"The secret of sticking to a diet," Dizzy said, "is discipline. If you have discipline, you can do anything."

Saxophonist and long-time friend Bill Schremp knew about Dizzy's discipline. "I've seen him take just one spoonful of ice cream at a banquet, when the rest of us were eating a bowlful," Schremp said.

Dizzy added, "I also exercise. I move around a lot. I walk fast."

That exuberance showed up early onstage in his clowning and pantomiming. It earned him that nickname, as celebrated as any in jazz history—"Dizzy."

Blowing His Own Horn

The enthusiasm also made him a good PR man. In Raymond Horricks's book *Dizzy Gillespie,* band member Quincy Jones recalls that while overseas, "Diz was always with cobras or camels or something for publicity purposes, but really, I think he enjoyed every minute of it, smoking an enormous meerschaum pipe or in Athens wearing full Greek national costume."

In his memoirs, *To Be or Not to Bop,* written with Al Frazer, Dizzy explained. "Comedy is important…when you're trying to establish audience control, the best thing is to make them laugh…. Sometimes I get up on the bandstand and say, 'I'd like to introduce the men in the band…' and then introduce the guys to one another." Dizzy found foreign audiences laughing at that one, too.

Dizzy always loved a good joke. In 1964, as a quasi-serious write-in presidential candidate, he hit the hustings with buttons, speeches, and a surprising amount of media attention. He even had his cabinet named—Peggy Lee as ministress of Labor; Ella Fitzgerald for Health, Education, and Welfare; Duke Ellington as Secretary of

State. And, of course, the White House would be renamed the Blues House.

But there was more to the Gillespie mystique than talent, technique, and showmanship. For one thing, there's that bent-bell trumpet.

It happened accidentally in 1953, at a birthday party for his wife, Lorraine. Two friends, fooling around, fell on the trumpet and bent the bell upward. Not wanting to make a fuss, Dizzy picked it up, played it, and liked the sound. After that he ordered all his trumpets with the bent bell. It was his trademark.

His other signature, the cheeks that ballooned out when he played, also "just happened" in mid-career. It began in the late '40s. It wasn't intentional. They just started looking like a frog when he played, he recalled. Although the pillows of air helped him build pressure for blowing, he didn't recommend them to young players.

South Carolina Start

Dizzy's own love of music started in his early days in Cheraw, South Carolina. He was playing a trumpet by the time he was 12.

Born John Birks Gillespie, October 21, 1917, Dizzy was ninth and last in a family in which seven children survived. James Gillespie, a strict father, died when Dizzy was 10, but his mother, Lottie, lived to 1959 and enjoyed her son's fame.

Dizzy had many memories of his boyhood. "I was always bad," he said. He remembers sticking gum in the girls' hair at school and whistling in the classroom when he was bored.

Dizzy may have been bad, but he was also smart. At 16, he won a music scholarship to the Laurinburg Institute in North Carolina. Two years later, he took off for Philadelphia, got a union card, and joined his first band.

Although his long career had its highs and lows, 1940 was a banner year. That's when he married dancer Lorraine Willis, whose down-to-earth advice and loyalty he credited with helping him become the musician he wanted to be. And that's the year he met Charlie "Yardbird" Parker, the musician who meant as much to him as any colleague he worked with.

That's saying a lot. The artists who populated Dizzy Gillespie's life re-create the American jazz scene that began in the late '30s. Louis Armstrong, Count Basie, Cab Calloway, Ray Charles, Miles Davis, Billy Eckstine, Duke Ellington, Ella Fitzgerald, Dexter Gordon, Lionel Hampton, Woody Herman, Billie Holiday, Thelonious Monk, and Sarah Vaughn are just a few.

He was quick to call himself a "musical descendent" of those who went before, and generous in giving credit to colleagues. Although the name "Dizzy Gillespie" is synonymous with be-bop, the musical craze that swept the country in the '40s, he asked that Charlie Parker be given the applause with him.

Bring On The Be-Bop

Dizzy named that new style by explaining the sound it made—"umpde-be-de-bop-be-bop."

If you wore a long coat, draped suit, and dark glasses in those days, you were called a "be-bopper." Gillespie, who always loved hats, sported a black beret and horn-rimmed glasses. They, too, became part of the be-bop look.

Dizzy's memoirs recall the first time Lionel Hampton heard Dizzy play be-bop. "It was entirely new, but it was so inventive. The harmonies, the chord structure, and the skill with which it was being played. He had a part where he jumped a couple of octaves. It just amazed me. I'd never heard a trumpet played that fast before," said Hampton.

By the late '40s, getting in touch with his strong feelings for his own African musical heritage, Dizzy added Afro-Cuban and Caribbean rhythms to America's musical center stage. "Jazz is close to South American music. They both had the same mother, Africa," he said.

And, lest you think he was not much of a businessman, there was his '50s Dee Gee record company, which allowed him to play both sides of the business.

By 1956 the government had taken official notice of jazz, and of Dizzy. The State Department asked him to be the first jazz musician to make an official overseas good-will tour. Dizzy loved it.

Through the years he was a regular on TV shows. Interviewed on the prestigious *Person to Person Show,* and a repeat guest on *The Tonight Show Starring Johnny Carson, Merv Griffin,* and *Today,* he also performed on *The Cosby Show.*

Besides such acknowledgments of his musical creativity, and his incomparable trumpet playing, Dizzy was a celebrated composer of songs like *Night in Tunisia, Manteca, Cubana Be Cubana Bop, Tin Tin Deo,* and *Con Alma.* At a White House concert, Dizzy coaxed President Jimmy Carter into a duet of another Gillespie number, *Salt Peanuts.*

Mr. Ambassador

Dizzy always did things his way. He never let age get in the way of his schedule. He was an ambassador not only for good music, but for good health. Dizzy admitted that there was one thing that could stop his nonstop lifestyle—poor health. He said, "I'm careful what I eat. I exercise. I'm not gaining weight. And I tell everybody, 'Ask the doctor about your diet, and do what he says. You don't want any of those bad surprises.'"

For Dizzy, life was always a blast.

Marcia Levine Mazur is senior editor of Diabetes Forecast.

Bill Davidson: Living the Family Legacy

by Marie McCarren

This article appeared in *Diabetes Forecast*, April 1994.

Bill Davidson knew what he wanted—had known since he was a kid. "At family functions," he says, "we were always talking motorcycles. It was something that I wanted to be involved in because it was a lot of fun. When you can combine your job with fun, you've got it made."

He was determined to make his career at Harley-Davidson, Inc., home of the all-American motorcycles. You might think that Davidson would have had no trouble landing a job there. After all, his great-grandfather founded the company. But in the early '80s, the Davidsons didn't control the purse strings, plus the company was laboring to come out of a slump and couldn't afford to be swayed by a name.

Davidson never assumed the family name would be enough. It's not in his nature to take things for granted. When he decides he wants something, he goes for it—but he goes prepared. He went to Harley-Davidson armed with a college degree (double major: marketing and finance), and he interviewed three times before landing the job.

Now, 10 years later, Davidson still has his dream job: During the day, he talks motorcycles, test drives motorcycles, works on improving motorcycles. Then he hops on his own motorcycle and goes home. And at the end of the week, he might take off somewhere for the weekend—yes, of course, on one of his motorcycles. "I'm a very fortunate man," he says. "My job is almost a hobby."

Davidson, 32, has been living and breathing motorcycles since—well, since he started living and breathing.

Growing up in a suburb of Milwaukee, Wisconsin, he was surrounded by Harley-Davidsons—the people and the bikes. His father, Willie G., has worked for the company for 31 years. His grandfather, William H., was president of the company from 1943 to 1973. And it all started with Bill's great-grandfather William A., who founded the company in 1903 with his brothers, Walter and Arthur, and William Harley.

Now a fourth generation of Davidsons has turned its passion for motorcycles into careers. Davidson's older sister, Karen, is in charge of fashion design at the company. Bill is product manager—a liaison between the customer and the company. He lets the people in the engineering and manufacturing departments know what features customers are asking for; he decides which models to produce and which ones to discontinue. "I've got the best of both worlds," Davidson says. "I'm giving input on the product, but I can still go out to the events and talk to the customers. I'm having the best time of my life."

Davidson is carrying on more than the family's motorcycle habit. Both of Bill's paternal great-grandparents developed diabetes as adults. So did Grandpa Davidson. Bill Davidson beat them by a mile—he developed diabetes before he was 3 years old.

Just Before His Third Birthday

Davidson's mom, Nancy, got concerned when young Bill started getting up at night to go to the bathroom. Her pediatrician didn't share her concern, but he told Nancy to drop off a urine sample to put her mind at ease.

Back home that same day, Bill got up from his afternoon nap and collapsed. While Nancy tried to rouse him, the pediatrician called with the results of the urine test and an urgent message: Get Bill to the hospital.

"My immediate reaction was just to get him some help, because he was close to comatose at the time," says Nancy. "The reality of it didn't set in for a few days."

Bill was in the hospital for 2 weeks. Although his blood glucose levels were under control, he couldn't go home until Nancy could show that she could give Bill his insulin shots. That was a roadblock she couldn't seem to pass—until she had a conversation in the hospital cafeteria.

"Every day I had coffee with another mother who had a child there," recalls Nancy. "We never discussed the children's problems, it was just a common thing—'oh, you have a child here'—so you felt some closeness there. Then one day she was in tears and blurted out the fact that her son was dying of cancer and she would never take him home.

"Of course with that I immediately went up to the nurse and said, I'm ready. I can give him the shot."

From then on, Nancy managed Bill's diabetes with matter-of-fact efficiency. "We were fortunate to have a wonderful doctor who got me on a strict routine," she says. "I just thought, 'This is the way it is.' I didn't know there was any room to be lax."

Bill learned the routine well, and when he was 8, he was ready to take over. He and his parents joined other families at the hospital for training. The parents went to a talk; the kids went to the lab, where they got the feel of giving an injection using syringes and oranges. "He came out of there just beaming," says Nancy.

"It was a big hurdle for me," recalls Davidson. "It was scary, but rewarding—that sense of control, of my responsibility."

Take a scary thing, get the proper training, and then do it. That's how the Davidsons approach what needs to be done—or what's destined to be.

At The Controls

Bill was 3 when he first rode on the back of his father's motorcycle. When he was 7, he moved up to the controls. "We had a motor home, and my family was going up north, camping. We had gotten the M50 [a 50 cc Harley-Davidson], and my father brought it with us. We stopped at a state park and he unloaded it and he said, 'Today's the day you're going to learn how to ride.' I was leaping I was so excited. I remember myself, my brother, and my sister all taking turns riding the M50."

His mother, who also rides, approved. "I wanted him to learn the right way," Nancy says, "and there was no better person to teach him than his father. The children had been around motorcycles since they were babies, so they had a great respect for them."

Davidson went on to race motorcycles through high school and into college. In motocross, as it's also called, the rider races around on a hilly, hard-packed dirt course of tight turns going up to 65 miles an hour, never sitting down. That activity did test the limits of his mother's enthusiasm, but Davidson insists it's a safe sport, in the right hands. He always dressed for safety, just as he routinely wears a helmet now whenever he's riding.

"You have to respect motorcycling: get the proper training, wear the protective gear, and be aware of your surroundings at all times. If you do those things, you can have fun with the sport and enjoy it for a lifetime."

Keeping control of a motorcycle is second nature to Davidson, just as managing his diabetes is.

"I have always been very strict with my routine. I believe that's one of the reasons I'm strong and healthy today.

"A lot of the credit goes to my folks and to my doctors. They made me realize the importance of the control—that it's not something that, if I don't do it, I'll notice now. But if I don't have the control now, down the road I could have problems."

Not a message all teenage boys would take seriously, and it did take a major spill to wake Davidson up to the wisdom of the words. He had a serious insulin reaction when he was in high school.

"During that time," says Davidson, "you're becoming an adult, you're experiencing new and different things, you're meeting new and more people, so it's easy to not be as concerned with the disease as you should be, and I think this happened to me."

A bout of the flu turned his control upside down, and Davidson ended up in the hospital in a coma.

"It made me realize that I am different, I do have something that I have to watch and control. I cannot neglect that. It said to me, Hey, your health is the most important thing in your life. It made me think about that, and stick to my strict routine."

When Davidson was a child, one shot a day and urine testing was typical diabetes management. When he was in high school, he heard about the new blood glucose monitoring systems, and got one as soon as they were available.

"The monitor has changed things drastically. Now you're truly your own doctor. You can fine-tune your control, which makes you feel better. You know what your system is doing, whereas before, you were on a path that was guided by instruments that weren't as specific as we have now. It has made a tremendous difference for me."

The only complication Davidson has had is some retinopathy. He had laser surgery on both eyes, and his eyes have been stable for 2 years now. "Thank God I had been going for eye checkups routinely, because they caught it at an early stage. I go in four times a year now, and they're very pleased with the results."

Regular exercise plays a big part in his diabetes management, and in his life. After talking to Davidson, you feel like you ought to run around the block, do a few dozen sit-ups, do something. His outside interests? Scuba diving, swimming, water skiing (he started when he was 5), and snowmobiling. Hobbies? He stills rides dirt bikes (though not competitively anymore) and enjoys skiing—both downhill and cross-country. And for actual exercise? Working out on his weight machine every day and riding a stationary bike.

Extended Families

When he's not under, on, or in water, or racing over snow, dirt, or the highway, Davidson fills his life with people. He's an extended-family man.

First, there is the community of bikers. It was his unofficial birthright to be a part of that community, but he also had an official role for almost 10 years. His first job at Harley-Davidson was as coordinator of the Harley Owners Group.

When you buy a Harley-Davidson motorcycle, you're automatically a member of the Harley Owners Group. HOG (Hog is also the nickname for a Harley-Davidson motorcycle) puts on events throughout the year and across the country. "It's much more than just a motorcycle," says Davidson. "There's the camaraderie, the fun, the socialization aspects of the sport."

He also gets that community feeling from other people who have diabetes. "There's camaraderie that exists among diabetics. You instantly have something in common, and you can talk about similar problems, bounce ideas off one another. There's a wealth of wanting to help one another and to try to find a cure."

Davidson, too, is hopeful of a cure, but it's not a high priority in his life. "If I didn't have to test my blood and give my injections, if I didn't have to worry about timing my food intake and my exercise, it would be strange for me. I've been brought up with it, and it's part of my life. If that disappeared I would maybe sense a little bit more freedom, but I don't feel a burden because of it now.

"But I do follow the research coming out. I want to make sure that if there's something that can help my control, I can look into that."

Davidson has recently taken on a more visible role in his second extended family—he joined the board of directors of the ADA Wisconsin Affiliate in August. He had worked with the affiliate in the past, organizing fundraising activities, and he is enjoying his more active role. "It's loads of fun, and I feel I'm giving more than in the past, which is rewarding for me."

Davidson plans to get his two communities together. "I'd love to develop some type of fundraising event where motorcycles and the people who ride them play a major role."

Will he ever get enough of motorcycling? Never, he says. "I have gasoline in my veins."

Marie McCarren is associate editor of Diabetes Forecast.

Zippora Karz: Toeing the Line

by Marcia Levine Mazur

This article appeared in *Diabetes Forecast,* May 1994.

You grow up fast in the world of ballet. That's why, at the age of 15, Zippora Karz had to make the decision of her life: go to college to teach deaf and blind children, or join the New York City Ballet (NYCB).

She hesitated, then embraced ballet, one of the world's most disciplined professions.

Wise Choice?

Sit for a minute in the massive New York State Theater at Lincoln Center and watch as the lights dim, the conductor raises his baton, and the gold curtain rises. Six lithe ballerinas in dazzling blue dresses flash across the stage, whirling, leaping, twisting, bending, their toes barely touching the floor.

There among them is Karz. Her dark hair, expressive hands, and swanlike neck tell you what she already knows. Yes, she chose wisely. Yes, she belongs here, among the soloists of the New York City Ballet, one of the world's premier dance companies.

Backstage, Karz, exotic in her flowing dress and flowered hairpiece, smiles and introduces herself.

But who can concentrate on amenities while dancers do knee-bends at an immense practice bar, or mill around unaware of the effect of their regal, straight-backed dancer's walk, or the way the stark backstage lighting highlights their wide-eyed makeup and splendid costumes?

Indeed, behind the scenes at Lincoln Center it's impossible to resist the pull of the near-fantasy world of professional ballet.

Sense Of Wonder

Karz still feels a sense of wonder at being there herself.

"Growing up in Northridge, California, I never had that little girl's dream of filmy tutus and satiny ballet shoes," she says.

Still, dancing was in her blood. Years earlier, her mother, Ellen Levand, had gone to New York to study modern dance. And she, too, had to make a decision: stay or leave.

She left.

Later, divorced and living in California, Levand enrolled her three daughters in ballet class so they could experience the joy of the dance. "It was beyond my wildest imagination that two would become professionals," Levand says.

(The oldest, Michele, dropped out of dancing. But Romy, the youngest, is now a member of the NYCB's *corps de ballet* and delighted that her sister is a soloist with the company.)

At first, Zippora Karz saw dancing as a joy, not a job, while an exceptional ballet teacher, Sheila Rosen, nurtured her talent.

But at age 13, the whole world seemed choreographed to put her on the stage. A scout from the San Francisco Ballet selected her for a summer of advanced training. One year later, the New York City Ballet invited her to their summer school, asked her back the following year, then invited her to stay.

One Chance

Karz knew what that meant: her one chance to join the NYCB. "Back then if you didn't get into their school before you were 16, you were considered too old," she explains.

She flew home and talked it over with her family, and 1 month later she was back in New York.

There, life was tough as well as thrilling. The special academic school she attended allowed time for practice and performances, but required extra hours to keep up with her academic workload.

Then there were the daily trips between school, home, and class. And always, there was the evening ballet to watch.

"I attended performances every night. It was incredible. I couldn't stay away. And that's when I knew I was in love with ballet," she says.

Captivated by the world of dance, Karz spent every available minute perfecting her art.

Three years later, that devotion began to pay off. She was promoted from the school to the company—one of four tapped from a class of nearly 100—and life grew even busier.

Crash

But 3 years after that, when Karz was 21, it all seemed to come crashing down. Frightening symptoms appeared: sores, then boils, developed under her arms where her costumes rubbed, and her already-svelte body seemed to be melting away.

She was stunned to learn that she had type 1 diabetes. "I had no idea what that meant, what I was dealing with," she recalls.

But the diagnosis prompted another question: How to keep dancing while maintaining good diabetes control?

"I knew I was never going to give up ballet, but I didn't know how to hold onto my career as well as my health," she recalls.

Once again, the Californian flew home to consult with her family, especially her father, Dr. Allen Karz, and her grandmother, Gloria Levand, who'd always had a special flair for healthy eating.

And that began Karz's battle to maintain the lightness, the exquisite elegance of her technique despite the diabetes. It wasn't easy. "I was terrified the disease would affect my dancing," she recalls.

On Her Toes

Her fear was well founded. To stay on her toes—literally—Karz has to make sure any pre-performance butterflies are nerves, not low blood glucose.

She faces another, unique, problem. "I'm a dancer. I have to feel the tips of my fingers and toes. If my sugar isn't right, I lose that vital connection."

To prevent that, Karz tests at least six times a day, and stashes a glucose meter backstage to use 15 minutes before curtain time, and during mid-dance costume changes. (The audience sees a smiling ballerina toeing into the wings. The dresser sees a hurried dancer grabbing for her glucose meter.)

She's got her diet figured out too. "I eat a lot, but I eat carefully," she explains. Karz limits herself to fruits, vegetables—especially an assortment of beans—free-range chickens, and all manner of grains. She uses winter squash or sweet potatoes to satisfy her sweet tooth.

The 5-foot-5, 105-pound ballerina munches a date when she needs a glucose boost because, she asks, "Why waste a calorie on sucrose?"

Karz makes no secret of her diabetes, and the management of the New York City Ballet is very supportive. So are her fellow performers. "They yell, 'Beam me up, Scotty,' when they hear my tester ping," she says, laughing.

For Karz, ballet continues to be a labor of joy. "We keep refining even the smallest technique," she explains, "the turnout of the leg, the line of the ankle, the position of the hips."

But her next sentence pops any illusion of the delicate ballerina. "What looks soft in us is actually rock hard. The audience sees us as graceful, but that is really the incredible strength in our feet. Our toes are like fingers. We can grip the floor through our shoes."

Karz, a realist, sees the dressing room she shares with several other ballerinas as "very unglamorous." No way. It's the stuff dreams are made of: make-up tables with mirrors circled by light bulbs, piles of pink ballet slippers, flowered hairpieces and sparkling crowns, false eyelashes, and even two bouquets on a tiny table. Unglamorous? It's a Hollywood vision of the ballet.

Broken Foot

But Karz admits there is a downside to this profession. Like athletes who push their bodies to the max, dancers are no strangers to physical breakdowns. Foot problems, especially infections, are common in the ballet world. And, again like athletes, dancers may seek professional help so they can perform even when they're not in top condition. "There's always a physical therapist on hand," Karz says, "because, the truth is, every day, everybody here has something hurting." And there's more.

"Once I came down from a jump and heard a pop, and I knew a bone was broken," she recalls. Her foot was in a cast for 6 weeks. For once, her timing was bad. Karz had been scheduled to perform in the film *George Balanchine's The Nutcracker,* but the accident forced her into a nondancing role.

Ballet slippers don't offer much protection from such breaks, either. In fact, Karz has some startling information about them. "Our shoes are made of cardboard. That's because we want them to hold their shape, but still be light, and not too noisy. The audience should never hear your shoes. I sometimes take a hammer and bang the tips of my shoes to soften the sound."

She adds, "You can see why we go through a pair or two of shoes a day. And by the end of a performance that pair is dead, too. We dance on our toes, so after awhile the tips get soft and don't give any support."

Although each performer's shoes are made to his or her exact specifications, the dancers themselves sew on the ribbons and elastic that hold the shoes to their feet. Karz adds an interesting tip. "We put resin on the toes of our tights to keep the foot from slipping inside the shoe."

Marathoners, Don't Apply

The New York City Ballet dancers have an exceptionally long schedule. They are in residence at Lincoln Center during both the winter and spring seasons, move to the Saratoga Performing Arts Center for 3 weeks in July, and may tour in August.

They also perform an astounding 50 ballets a season, with each dancer doing perhaps four or five different ballets a week.

How does Karz remember all the steps?

"If it's good choreography, your body remembers," she explains. "That's what's so wonderful about Balanchine's dances. Once he put steps to music it seems like only those steps could go with that music. Martins [Ballet Master-in-Chief Peter Martins] is very supportive of the way Balanchine worked. And when the choreography is that good, your feet know what to do."

Karz's schedule would shame a marathoner. Six days a week she begins with an hour-and-a-half warmup class, then a 2- or 3-hour rehearsal for a future ballet, an hour on the evening's performance, with yet another rehearsal for a ballet still being created. "Every day is a little different," she adds.

Conscious of her diabetes, Karz makes sure she takes time out for dinner, but that allows her muscles to get cold. What then? Another 45 minute practice session before she tests her glucose, ties on her ballet slippers, and steps onstage.

Standing On Her Own Feet

Today, all the parts of Karz's world have come together. Last spring, at age 27, she was selected one of the 15 soloists of the company's 100-plus members. (Soloists occupy the level between *corps de ballet* and principal dancer.) And her star is still rising.

"I do everything in my power to stay healthy," she says. "I take my disease in my own hands, and I thoroughly believe in tight control."

But there are occasional doubts. "The work, the pain, the effect on my body, especially with the diabetes…I sometimes wonder, 'Is the ballet really worth it?' And then I have one of those magical moments onstage, a moment so beautifully fulfilling, so satisfying, that it dissolves my doubts and makes it all worthwhile."

Marcia Levine Mazur is senior editor of Diabetes Forecast.

Kent Thompson and Tim Langan: Sugar-Free Shakespeare

by Marcia Levine Mazur

This article appeared in *Diabetes Forecast,* February 1993.

Lights dim, the curtain rises, and a hush falls over the audience. It's opening night at the Alabama Shakespeare Festival, and offstage, Kent Thompson and Tim Langan are following every scene. As the final act winds to a close, they eagerly await the audience response. Will the rafters shake with applause? Have they got a success? If past is truly prologue, the answer is yes. No wonder. At the ASF Kent Thompson and Tim Langan are helping power one of the most prestigious regional theaters in America. They play different roles, though. Thompson, the artistic director, is the man to see if you want an audition. Langan, the managing director, will tell you how much you'll earn if you make it.

But the two share more than a love of theater. Each has type 1 diabetes. That quirk of fate provided them with a pet name for the festival: Sugar-Free Shakespeare.

What's In A Name?

But if "sugar-free" doesn't really describe this spectacular theater complex in Montgomery, Alabama, neither does its official name, the Alabama Shakespeare Festival.

True: ASF plans to mount all of Shakespeare's 37 plays in an 8-year cycle (*A Midsummer Night's Dream* and *Henry IV, Parts I and II,* this season.)

But it also offers classics by Chekov, Ibsen, and Shaw; American standards (*Our Town* and *Raisin in the Sun* in '93); and new plays by Southern writers.

There are rollicking Broadway musicals, too, currently *Big River*. And the international Piano Masters Series. If you plan it right, you can visit Montgomery for the weekend and take in four shows.

The ASF isn't quite a festival, either. That implies a limited season, but this theater is lit from November until August, with plans to operate year-round.

(There is a festival, though, from March through July. Come then, and take in *six* plays in one weekend.)

Keeper Of The Purse

Ah, but who thinks of numbers as Romeo climbs Juliet's balcony, Hamlet asks whether to be or not to be, or Marc Antony comes to bury, not to praise, Caesar?

Actually, Tim Langan does. "I'm like the business executive of a company," he explains. "At the ASF I manage a budget just under $6 million, which means I get to say, 'Yes, we can,' or 'No, we can't afford it.'"

Langan took over as ASF's managing director in 1991 after 11 years in that same chair at the Trinity Repertory Company in Providence, Rhode Island.

He grew up loving theater. "Susan Hayward is my dad's first cousin," he explains. "Her real name is Edith Marrener and she was named after my grandmother Edith, who helped support her when she went to Hollywood."

Langan averages about 60 hours a week on the job, teaching graduate courses in theater, talking to local groups, and traveling the country promoting the ASF.

Churning Stress

Eight years ago Langan developed diabetes. It happened just after he had passed his 32nd birthday and had made it through one of the most exciting but difficult years of his life.

During that time he held a tension-filled job, was newly married, and experienced instant fatherhood (his wife had two daughters by a previous marriage). In the midst of all these changes, he met with sudden grief. Just 10 days after he was married, Langan's father died. And there was more.

The couple bought a new house, ran into financial difficulties, and almost went bankrupt. Then, during their first week in the new house, one of Langan's daughters became seriously ill. (She's doing fine now.)

"The stress was always churning inside of me," he recalls.

Langan noticed his weight loss and constant thirst but didn't pay much attention. He only knew he was winning the bet he and his wife, Pat, had made: The first to lose 10 percent of his or her weight would choose the couple's next antique.

Although Tim was clearly losing more than Pat, he didn't know why. After all, he was still digging into his morning doughnut and gulping six soft drinks a day.

He also noticed that, while he used to be able to drive from Florida to Pennsylvania without needing a bathroom, he could no longer make it from Boston to New York.

"I found the symptoms merely interesting," he recalls, "until the night I wet the bed." That drove him to the doctor.

Thompson: Getting Into The Act

If possible, Kent Thompson, the theater's artistic director, spends even more time on the job than Langan. Besides traveling, auditioning new talent, and consulting at other theaters, he attends most rehearsals.

"I am responsible for everything that happens onstage," he says. "I decide what plays we are going to do, hire designers, composers, dialect coaches, even choreographers for fight scenes. I see that we have sets, clothes, lights, and sound. Typically, I also direct four or five shows a year, which keeps me in rehearsals 42 to 47 hours a week."

Thompson, who came to ASF in 1989, spent the previous 10 years as a freelance director at professional theaters throughout the country and in Canada.

Diagnosis: Ulcers

But at age 33, Thompson discovered more drama offstage than on.

"It was the end of my first season at the festival," he recalls. "I was in a new job and a new place, and I was going through the waiting period all directors go through to see how their work turns out. And, coincidentally, I had gotten married 2 weeks after I took the job."

Then came weight loss, thirst, and frequent urination. "I thought it was the heavy work and travel load," he recalls. "Then I developed bad stomach pains, so I wasn't surprised when a doctor prescribed ulcer medication."

But it didn't help.

One night Thompson felt so sick his wife, Carol, had to rush him to the emergency room. That's where he learned the difficulty wasn't ulcers, but diabetes.

Symptoms of unregulated diabetes are behind both men, but long hours, travel, and job stress are not.

All The World's A Stage

At times, ASF resembles a medieval village.

"When we are fully producing a show, there are crafts people here making everything from jewelry and armor to sets, costumes, and shoes. They also stencil, silk screen, applique, and dye fabrics, when necessary," Thompson says.

(ASF sells everything it can't reuse or rent out. Buyers often put whole sets in their yards or living rooms; Macbeth's severed head sells every time.) There is also a cadre of actors and their families who live nearby for half a year or so as part of the resident acting company. The late Tony Award winner, Cleavon Little, was one such ASF resident.

As You Like It

You can't mention the Alabama Shakespeare Festival without sighing over its idyllic setting.

The complex—the Carolyn Blount Theater housing the 750-seat Festival Stage and the smaller 225-seat Octagon—sits on a landscaped esplanade overlooking a placid lake.

The park is named for its benefactor, businessman and former U.S. Postmaster General Winton M. Blount. His astonishingly generous gift to the ASF, $21.5 million, is probably the largest single donation in the history of the American theater.

Because the Alabama climate is so temperate, the park's rolling lawn and scattered trees always seem lush with summer greenery or splashed in rich autumn colors. (Stroll through the park some balmy afternoon, and you might come across Tim Langan teaching his classes outdoors.)

For Thompson, the picture is described by many a first-time visitor's response to the view. "It comes when they enter the park, turn the corner, and suddenly, across the lake, they spot the theater. We call it the 'Oh God' moment," Thompson says.

Perchance To Dream

But the ASF's program isn't as relaxed as its setting. Behind the scenes, this theater is always alive with new ideas. Right now Thompson is cultivating its regional roots by promoting Southern writers. (They may soon mount a two-play epic on LBJ by bestselling author John Jakes.)

"Look at the great writers the South has produced," Langan adds. "I think it's because the people here love—absolutely love—storytelling."

The theater also wants to bring more of its neighbors into the act. The Lila Wallace–*Reader's Digest* grant they've received will help fund a program to encourage more African Americans to attend productions and join the staff.

What Of Diabetes?

Any qualms that diabetes will interfere with ambition? Not at all.

"It has taken me a long time to realize that half of doing a good job is taking care of yourself," Thompson says. "But it's difficult. The theater is so labor intensive, and virtually every lunch is a working one."

He has managed to change his routine, however. "Monday is my day off," he says, "and even though I have thousands of deadlines a year, diabetes has taught me to drop them out of my mind, and take Monday off."

Langan seems to be reading from the same script. "This is a particularly challenging profession to be in and have diabetes," he says. "I used to work 7 days and nights a week. I would come in at 9 o'clock in the morning, and then on my way home I'd pick up a pizza and watch *The Tonight Show*. I had to figure out how to work smarter, because I sure couldn't work longer."

He adds, "I can't emphasize how important a good attitude is. And for me, part of that attitude is not leaving the management of my disease to others. I have to stay involved."

Both Langan and Thompson give a standing round of applause to their wives, Pat and Carol, for keeping them on track nutritionally.

The ASF staff is also on their team. "We installed a juice machine, as well as a new refrigerator so they could keep fruit in it," says Sarah Findlay, director of press and public relations for ASF.

Diabetes Times Two

Working with someone else who has diabetes seems to be "a dream devoutly to be wished." It has certainly made things easier for Langan and Thompson. "I find it helpful to our professional partnership because we both understand that, as demanding as the job is, we must take care of ourselves," Thompson says.

"I am blessed to have a partner who understands," echoes Langan. "I used to be embarrassed to leave a meeting because I had to get something to eat. Not anymore."

On occasion, the men borrow each other's testing equipment, or remind each other that it's time for a snack.

"On our first trip to New York together it got to be 2 or 3 in the afternoon and we were getting pretty cranky," Thompson recalls. "Then we both realized how stupid we'd been. We hadn't eaten lunch and we had low blood sugars."

Neither had to explain why they immediately sat down for a snack.

Marcia Levine Mazur is senior editor of Diabetes Forecast.

Bobby Clarke: Skating at the Cutting Edge

by Leslie Y. Dawson

This article appeared in *Diabetes Forecast,* March 1994.

Robert Earle Clarke was 3 years old when he first hit the ice, hockey stick in hand, in his family's backyard skating rink in Flin Flon, Manitoba, Canada. Today, more than 40 years later, he's known to millions of hockey fans as Bobby Clarke, captain of the Philadelphia Flyers during their heyday in the 1970s.

Now Clarke watches hockey from a box—the general manager's box. Since March 1, 1993, he's been general manager and vice president of the Miami Panthers, the latest National Hockey League expansion team in the Atlantic Division. (He came to the Miami team after serving as general manager for the Flyers, the Minnesota North Stars, and the 1987 Team Canada.) Clarke is now in the business of bringing talent—and hockey—to the tropics.

Trading Skates For Roller Blades

Nine years after retiring from active professional play, Clarke is still remembered as one of the baddest of the bad of the Philadelphia Flyers' legendary Broad Street Bullies. This hockey dynasty presented the city of Philadelphia with its first Stanley Cup in 1973–74, followed by another in 1974–75. Those two spectacular seasons cured the city of a gloomy self-image as a perpetual loser. When the Flyers won the cup, 2 million crazed fans flooded Broad Street to celebrate. Other fans honored Clarke by showing up at his residence and "streaking" the premises. (To those of you not familiar with fads of the 1970s, streaking refers to running around naked.)

Clarke had one boyhood dream: to win the Stanley Cup. He counts the actual experience of winning it—twice—as among the greatest moments of his life. Skating around the rink, flaunting that gleaming trophy to adoring, screaming fans…that was "it." Later, winning against the Russian national team with Team Canada was "a bonus."

In 1993, the Flyers' stat sheet still ranked Clarke as their all-time leading offensive player. He racked up leading numbers for points (1,210) (points combine number of goals plus number of assists); assists (852) (a pass to a player who then scores a goal); games played (1,144); and shorthanded goals (32) (goals scored while a player is missing due to penalty). He's also their all-time top rookie scorer (in 1969). Clarke still ranks fourth for Flyer penalty minutes (1,453), and in the top 10 for goals (358), overall center performance, power-play goals (99) (scored while the opposing team is shorthanded), and hat tricks (5) (scoring three goals in one game).

For most of his life, Clarke could not imagine a life without the daily pursuit of a black puck skidding across the ice in excess of 100 miles per hour. "For me, playing the game of hockey was everything," Clarke recalls. "If I could have held my age stationary at 23, I would have."

But Clarke could not make time stand still. "If you're an athlete, you know you only have so many years on the job," he says. His stretch was impressive; he played professionally for 15 years, and as an amateur for another 19.

When he retired from active play, Clarke experienced a sharp sense of loss. But he also felt challenged to find another place for himself in the world of hockey. Now he's playing, very intensely, in that arena again. But from another position, of course.

Clarke, 45, says he finds great satisfaction in working with his new team. "I'm still involved in the outcome of games," he explains. Although he no longer wears the skates, it's *his* players on the ice, and the game matters as much to him as it ever did.

Clarke says he put on skates only once this winter. Instead, three or four times a week, he dons roller blades

after supper and pours on the speed around a lake in sub-
urban Miami.

Another Sort Of Courage

What hockey stat sheets do not reveal about Clarke is
his probable status as the first professional hockey player to
have diabetes—at least the first one to go public with it.
The only recognition he received for this aspect of his
game came in 1980, when Philadelphia sportswriters honored him with their Most Courageous Athlete Award. The
sportswriters noted that he coped so well with diabetes that
most people in the world of sports came to ignore it.

At the time the award was given, *Philadelphia Daily News*
sportswriter Ted Silary wrote: "Bobby Clarke, great hockey
player, looms large enough. Bobby Clarke, great player
and conqueror of diabetes, is almost too much, especially
for him."

It would have been hard for Clarke to imagine receiv-
ing this award when, at the age of 13, he was diagnosed
with type 1 diabetes. The news came as a terrible shock to
the boy; there had been no diabetes in his family for several generations. "I don't remember too much, but I had the
normal symptoms—weight loss, excessive thirst. I was hos-
pitalized," he recalls.

Young men growing up in Flin Flon could choose
between two livelihoods: hockey and hardrock mining.
Bobby's dad worked the mines. When Clarke was diagnosed with diabetes, hockey was still foremost in his mind.
He had already logged 10 years on the ice.

Clarke's first question to his doctor was asked in des-
peration: "Will I be able to continue playing hockey?"

"Yes, I would, he told me," Clarke recalls.

That fact established, he and his family set about learning as much as they could about diabetes. In those days, the
routine included boiling syringes and weighing food por-
tions. Because he was so active in hockey, Clarke was
allowed a higher-than-normal number of calories.

Only twice in all the years he played hockey did Clarke's
blood sugars go dangerously low. Once, in Junior Hockey
Camp, he was playing an afternoon game and didn't rec-

ognize the symptoms of hypoglycemia (low blood sugar) coming on. The team doctor did, however, and walked him across the street to a conveniently located hospital.

A more serious incident took place on Clarke's first day of Pro Camp. He overslept. Anxious not to be late for practice, he skipped breakfast. Later, on the way home, crowded into a car with teammates, he collapsed. His teammates, aware of his diabetes, took him into the hospital. There, he was treated intravenously, most likely with glucagon. "The doctor gave me a lecture and let me go," he recalls.

Despite the fact that he has never had another such incident, Clarke still carries glucose tablets with him as a precaution. He is also better at identifying the symptoms of hypoglycemia.

Early in his career, Clarke simply would not discuss diabetes with sportswriters, whom he felt did not properly understand the disease. "I didn't like being called 'the diabetic hockey player.' I was a hockey player who had diabetes," he says.

Some fans of opposing teams also had a poor grasp of the disease, and some attempted to taunt Clarke because of his condition. Silary recalls that "loonies in New York's Madison Square Garden threw packets of sugar onto the ice." Clarke recalls a time when "loudmouth Penguins' fans" would try to entice him with chocolate bars—as if eating candy would cripple his performance.

Clarke was among the first to use modern blood glucose testing equipment. "One advantage of being a professional athlete is that you get the new technology before anyone else," he says. Clarke says his blood glucose runs between 120 and 130 milligrams per deciliter (mg/dl). He credits his good control to exercise. He runs 5 to 10 miles every morning. (He started a daily running routine when he was 16.) He lifts weights and skates on roller blades three times a week. "I'm a real firm believer in lots of exercise," he says.

Clarke also enjoys golf, although he describes himself as an "average" duffer. Clarke loves the game's personal challenge—he especially loves competing against himself. It's ironic, but since he's moved to Florida, golfer's heaven, Clarke has been too busy to play golf.

On Fighting

Clarke's intense drive to win fueled his reputation as an ice fighter. Winning is "what you get paid for," he explains. Clarke's attitude toward hockey violence flies in the face of that expressed by many observers of the scene today.

Clarke believes that physical confrontations are an essential part of the game. "Three or four guys are fighting to get the puck in the corner. You're slashing at them and they're slashing at you. That's enjoyable."

Concerning recent proposals to eliminate hockey fighting and even body-checking, he adds derisively, "That's when they'll make it figure skating. It's a physical sport."

Fortunately for Clarke, he was never seriously injured in a hockey fight or play. (A "serious" injury, he notes, is when a joint or bone is damaged. He considers other injuries, such as cuts, bruises, and lost teeth, to be "a small price to play for the privilege of playing hockey.")

In contrast to his rough reputation against other teams, Clarke made a career out of teamwork and sacrificing personal goal-scoring glory for assists. His career total for assists stands a universe above those of his former teammates. Next in line to his 852 assists is Brian Propp, with 480. Says Clarke, "I'd just as soon set a goal up as get the goal."

Moderation In An Immoderate World

Clarke credits diabetes with educating him about nutrition. For instance, as a young athlete, he learned how to manage carbohydrates in his diet.

"I don't eat a perfectly balanced diet, with all the exchanges, but I'm not an overeater or a compulsive eater," he says. "I have a lot better diet now than before I got diabetes. People didn't eat as healthy back then."

Clarke, who joined the Panthers at the invitation of team owner Wayne Huizenga, finds that life in hockey management presents a great deal more stress than he felt in his playing days.

"I felt no stress at all on the ice," says the man once infamous for his fierce play. "But at the management level, things get out of your control and start to affect you. For instance, say two players get injured and that will affect the next three games...." Since joining the Panthers, Clarke has signed many players through the professional and amateur drafts. He has also signed former New York Ranger coach Roger Neilson, and ex-Ranger goaltender John Vanbiesbrouck. Clarke has not set point goals for his team's first season, but he has set high expectations. "I expect the guys are going to work hard, and if they don't, we'll pull someone up from the minor leagues who will."

Team spokesman Greg Bouris said that Clarke has recruited the Panthers "in his own image." The core of Clarke's team is half-a-dozen experienced "character players," led by Vanbiesbrouck. The rest of the 20-man squad is made up of younger skaters led by 19-year-old center Rob Niedermayer. Bouris calls the fledgling team "scrappy, hard-checking, and intense."

Just like Clarke.

Leslie Y. Dawson is a freelance writer and a former editor at ADA.

Audrey Broussard Welcomes You to Cajun Country

by Marcia Levine Mazur

This article appeared in *Diabetes Forecast,* February 1996.

Come listen to a love story that echoes through two centuries.

It begins in the early 1700s, in a land called Acadia in today's Canadian province of Nova Scotia. There, two brothers, Joseph and Alexander Beau de Soleil Broussard, married two sisters, Agnes and Marguerite Thibodeaux.

But they did not live happily ever after.

Some years after the weddings, they, their children, and all the people of French Acadia were forced from their land and herded onto British ships. Victims of the French and British grab for New World land, the bewildered, fearful, and destitute Acadians were deposited in ports along the Atlantic Seaboard.

Families were separated; out of a population of 18,000, half died, and 7,000 more became refugees.

Although some Acadians wandered for years, many eventually found their way to Southern Louisiana.

There, rallying around home, family, and church, they established closeknit farming and fishing communities. And there, to preserve their culture, they settled in near isolation along the bayous (waterways), marshes, and prairies of Southern Louisiana.

There, too, in a mispronunciation of the name of their Acadian homeland, they came to be called Cajuns.

Most survived and prospered.

Not so for the Beau de Soleil Broussards. One year after they landed, Joseph, Agnes, Alexander, and

Marguerite were dead of a fever contracted in the sub-tropics of Louisiana.

Yet today their descendants, the Broussards, form the bulk of one of the largest Cajun families in Louisiana.

And what about the love story? In its own way, it lived on too. J. Maxie Broussard—descendant of Joseph and Agnes—fell in love with Audrey Broussard—descendant of Alexander and Marguerite—and in 1953, they married.

But unlike their forebears, Audrey Broussard can say, "If you want to find *joie de vivre*—the joy of life—come see us."

The "us" are the modern Cajuns of Southern Louisiana.

Typical

Besides enjoying a *joie de vivre,* Audrey and Maxie are typical of their people in other ways. They grew up speaking French at home, prize good food, maintain a close family life, and lean on their Catholic faith.

But there are two other ways that Audrey is also representative of her community; she carries excess weight, and she has type 2 diabetes, a disease that is widespread among the Cajuns.

Although Audrey was diagnosed at age 40, she had been expecting diabetes for years.

Both her mother's brother, Nathan, and her own brother, Rodney, had uncontrolled type 2 diabetes, and each died of a heart attack in his early 50s. Her mother's sister, Nita Trahan Bourque, as well as Maxie's grandmother, Bertha Baudoin Simon, each had a leg amputated because of the disease. Diabetes caused Audrey's mother to lose her sight in the last 6 months of her life.

Up-To-Date Care

Today, while diabetes remains a stark feature of the Cajun landscape, the Cajuns are learning to understand and deal with it. In fact, the Cajuns of old would never recognize the diabetes regimen Audrey follows to keep her type 2 diabetes under control.

Audrey Broussard monitors her blood glucose and takes insulin injections daily; she sees her medical doctor as well as her eye doctor and dentist regularly.

She has her blood pressure read often, has her feet checked every 4 weeks, and wears closed-toe shoes, even in summer. "My friends with diabetes have problems with their toes. I want to make sure that doesn't happen to me," she explains. She also attends American Diabetes Association classes held in nearby Lafayette.

"But the real difficulty," Audrey concludes, "is food. I'm 5 foot 4 inches tall. Although I'm big-boned like most of the Cajuns, I weighed 205 pounds when I was diagnosed. I went to exercise classes for a year and a half, and I've come down to 179 pounds."

Cherie Heslop, a registered dietitian and a Cajun herself, sums up the problem. "Food is like a second religion to the Cajuns."

Audrey and Maxie prove the point. They are open-handed hosts, welcoming family and guests with cups, bowls, plates, and platters of steaming crawfish etouffee, fricasse, chicken piquante, gumbos, stews, andouille sausage, and all manner of other pork dishes.

They even put up a full second kitchen in an old farm building in the back of their house.

When company is expected, Maxie stirs up ample servings of old favorites in a big black jambalaya pot that's been in the family for years.

It's no surprise that the abundance of the spicy, mouth-watering Cajun cuisine is difficult for Audrey to resist. But she is doing well, and practices low-fat cooking methods she learned at ADA-sponsored cooking demonstrations.

A Farmer's World

Audrey's world, like her medical care, is a far cry from the one she once knew.

"I was raised in a small town called Andrew, about 150 miles from New Orleans," she recalls.

"We were all Cajun there and only about half the people spoke English. In fact, if someone spoke English well, or didn't go to the Catholic church, we called them "American." We all went to school together in a small town called Indian Bayou. That's how Maxie and I met.

"My daddy Edlar had what we'd call a grocery store but

they called it a general merchandise store back then. He was the postmaster because the post office was inside the store.

"Maxie's family had a dairy farm, so he took a degree in dairy husbandry from Southwestern Louisiana University in Lafayette. We brought up our children—Brenda (a registered dietitian and a certified diabetes educator), John, Byron, and Debra—on the farm. We raised everything we ate, even chicken, beef, and hogs," Audrey recalls.

"And we grew wonderful vegetables. I still relish those moist sweet potatoes baked in their jackets. We ate what we call cous-cous and milk for breakfast. That's whole kernels of corn ground into a kind of meal, not a flour. We would wet the meal, salt it, and fry it in a heavy skillet. We only bought maybe rice and flour."

Today, Audrey runs a bed-and-breakfast on the remodeled 160-year-old farm. She loves hosting her stream of French-speaking guests, but is equally pleased that couples from Texas return again and again.

Her table may be part of the reason. "We have an orchard and I make fig, peach, pear, and blackberry jellies. But I don't bake my own bread anymore. There's a French bakery nearby now and I buy it there."

Welcome

Cajun people are friendly. They welcome the world to their towns and festivals. Still, there is an insular, closed quality to this community.

Maxie explains it this way. "We are extremely friendly to strangers, but still clannish. If you are Cajun and you meet another Cajun, he will ask you who your father and your grandfather were. Those attitudes are not erased even in a few generations.

"And when a guy from, say, a German background marries into a French family here, he becomes French, no matter what."

Festivals

Nothing defines the Cajuns so much as their love of festivals. Their sheer joy of life bursts out then. As Audrey puts it, "We just love to have a good time!"

Still, when thousands throng to New Orleans for the Mardi Gras parade, people like Audrey and Maxie are not among them.

"We prefer to celebrate Mardi Gras in our own towns," Audrey explains. "It's safer and quieter. And it's more meaningful. After all, Ash Wednesday begins at midnight the night of Mardi Gras—Mardi Gras means Fat Tuesday—and that Wednesday is the beginning of Lent," she explains.

For Audrey, autumn is the best time of year. The fall festivals come on then, weekend after weekend, in town squares and fairgrounds all around the parishes (counties) of Cajun country.

Excitement crackles through the air as large families gather together for the rice, shrimp, and sugar cane festivals. There seems no end of good times, including the Festival de Musique Acadienne, Bayou Food Festival, Louisiana Native Crafts Festival, and the Festival International de Louisiane for starters.

People march in parades and enjoy the craft displays while accordianists send the old French tunes echoing across the village square. And when the fiddles and triangles strike up the Cajun and Zydeco (snap bean) rhythms, everyone—young and old—swings onto the dance floor.

And always there is food, food, food. It may be washed down with beer, but rarely hard liquor.

The Cajun men, among the world's best cooks, man the huge black cook pots, passed down for generations, and proudly mix in "just another pound of sausage."

"Folks come from miles to savor Maxie's jambalaya," Audrey adds.

A New Life

However, while the festivals remain, much of the Cajun world is rapidly changing. Audrey's grandmother—Elise Duhon Trahan—had 15 children, while Audrey has had 4. "We don't have such large families anymore, and that is a good thing," Audrey says.

And, where Elise's generation rarely strayed far from home and often cared little for education—Elise could not read or write—today's Cajuns are heading for college in record numbers.

That has put a damper on another tradition, widespread intermarriage. Many members of the younger generation now take spouses from other regions of the country, and for Audrey that too, is a good thing.

"There used to be a lot of inbreeding. You would meet a Cajun and find out he was a distant cousin," she recalls. "That wasn't healthy for our children."

Still, such changes are writing *fini* to a unique culture. Many children of this community—the largest concentration of French-speaking people in the United States—no longer know the language.

But take heart. There is still moonlight on the bayou, and sunrise over the lush Atchafalaya Swamp. You can still order fresh crawfish, yams, red beans and rice, or alligator sauce piquante in roadside restaurants in Cajun country. And—if you listen hard—you'll still catch the beat of homemade Cajun music played on spoons or a wooden washboard.

Marcia Levine Mazur is senior editor of Diabetes Forecast.

Mark Collie: Roadhouses and Revivals

by Marie McCarren

This article appeared in *Diabetes Forecast,* June 1995.

Mark Collie cut his teeth on rock, but country kept calling.

You can't do it. You can't slap Mark Collie's latest CD, *Unleashed,* in your stereo, crank up "Hard Lovin' Woman," and *not start* playing air guitar in the middle of your living room.

If you don't think it sounds 100 percent country, you're not alone. Depending on which song they're talking about, critics have described Collie's music as rockabilly, pop-rock, country-rock, country-soul, Memphis soul, and R&B. "Shame Shame Shame Shame," one of the hits from his third album, was called doo-wop.

Hey, that's what country music is today. "It's not exactly the country music that your mama and daddy listened to," says Collie. "We're an evolution of what's gone on before. We're all influenced by John Fogarty, John Lennon, and Johnny Cash, too."

But Collie stands out even in the varied pack that makes up country music today. Shannon Parks, from *Country Weekly* magazine, says Collie has a different look and a different sound, and she predicts it's going to keep him popular long after others are forgotten. "Mark doesn't wear the hat, the belt buckle, the boots, and the pressed jeans and white shirt," she says. "He's funky; he lets his creativity show.

"And he doesn't sound like everybody else. His music has the country feel and beat, but it's not typical. It's got a blues edge, sometimes hard rock. He's built a niche for himself."

The staple of country music is the love song, and Collie has contributed his share. 'Course, it is country, so you gotta have a little pain in your love songs. "Even The Man In The Moon Is Cryin'" (if that isn't sad, what is?), from Collie's third album, was a No. 2 hit.

"I think sad songs make us feel better," says Collie. "It's like sad movies. Everybody comes out weeping and says, 'I just loved that movie.' It reassures us that we're human and that we're not alone. I think that's what music does, and it does it at a lot of levels."

Don't Touch That Guitar!

Collie, 39, has been writing songs and playing guitar since he was 8. You could say his older brother, Steve, helped launch his career. "Steve was the first guy in the family to get a guitar," Collie recalls. "He told my brother John and me that if we ever touched the guitar, he'd kill us. So when he'd leave, the first thing we'd do was get the guitar out. It's a good way to teach someone to play. Buy an instrument and say 'never touch this.'"

Collie started by just "banging it out." When he got around guitarists, he'd get them to show him a note here, a chord there, a lick or two. Soon the young Collie was entertaining at family get-togethers in Waynesboro, Tennessee.

As he got better, he played at local dances with his sister's future husband, Clark Rose, who is his road manager today. "Clark helped me a lot," says Collie. "I sang in gospel quartets with him. Then during the week, I'd work for his daddy hauling hay."

When he was in high school, Collie would slip off to the Tennessee-Alabama state line and play at the beer joints there. "It was more rock 'n' roll than it was country music in those days, because people in the bars and clubs weren't dancing to country music as much as they are now."

Yet Collie sang in church, too. "It was strange. I would be singing in the roadhouses on Saturday night and then playing the revivals on Sunday afternoon. Many a Sunday I felt like the preacher was speaking directly to me."

Getting Serious

For all the time he was putting into it, Collie was still just playing at the music game. "I rarely recorded the songs that

I wrote," he says. "Many I didn't even write down. I don't want to try to remember how many songs I wrote and forgot."

Partly it was youth, and maybe partly it was the diagnosis of diabetes that came when he was 20.

"I was a lousy patient," Collie says. "First it was the 'why me, Lord' stage. Then I thought, well if I do have this disease, it's probably going to kill me anyway, so I'm going to have a lot of fun before it does. So I was rather reckless, and I used the disease as an excuse to be that way."

At that time, people did urine testing to monitor their blood glucose levels. Collie said some days he'd do a test, other days he wouldn't, and he often had reactions.

Shortly after he was diagnosed, Collie was in Iran just before the overthrow of the Shah, touring with a U.S.O. show. (Collie had considered joining the Air Force, in keeping with family tradition, but diabetes nixed that plan. Playing in U.S.O. shows got him as close as he could get.)

Driving from the airport to the base, he had a serious insulin reaction and collapsed. "When I woke up, I was in a hospital in the middle of the desert, and the Dutch missionaries were giving me last rites, asking me if I knew Jesus Christ," he recalls.

"They left me there all afternoon. I was lying there, and two of the guys from the band came over to see me. They snuck me out of the hospital, and I performed that night."

His wife, Anne, who met Collie during that time, confirms he was a "wild child." But she admits, "We were both kind of wild."

Father And Serious Musician

Those reckless ways eventually lost their luster. "One day," says Collie, "I woke up, and I was 25 years old, and I felt like hell. I thought, well, I could live a long time, but I don't want to feel like this my whole life.

"I realized what a foolish and ignorant way of life that was, and that if I was going to be in the music business and write songs, I should be more serious about it. And meeting Anne about that time helped give me a direction."

The Collies, who by then were living in Memphis, soon had to do a lot of growing up together. Their son, Nathan, was born 2 months premature. Struggling artists rarely have good insurance coverage, and those with diabetes have an even harder time getting covered. As the medical bills piled up, Collie considered giving up on music. But Anne wouldn't let him.

"It wasn't a case of love being blind," she says. "He had the talent."

Anne is a painter, but two starving artists in one family is one too many, so Anne got a steady job while Collie kept on with his music. She supported the family working as a retouch artist. ("Ten pounds and 10 years removed instantly," is how Collie puts it.) Much of her work can be seen on album covers coming out of Nashville.

Finally, "Even The Man In The Moon Is Cryin,'" which Collie wrote with Don Cook, hit the charts. The days of scraping by were over for the Collies.

Racing Toward A Cure

With his career on track, Collie has been able to focus some energy on diabetes—his own and others'.

"After Nathan was born, I realized I had to stay healthy for him and Anne," he says. "I'd go to my doctor's office and see another diabetic. Then I'd see that same person again in 6 months, and he had lost a couple of toes.

"It started hitting home that this disease is killing people and is devastating lives, and it could do the same to me. I began to read more about diabetes, be more focused, and keep a closer check on it."

When Collie heard the results of the Diabetes Control and Complications Trial (DCCT), which proved that tight control of blood glucose levels slows or prevents the long-term complications of diabetes, he went on intensive insulin therapy. He takes 3 to 4 shots a day and tests his blood at least 8 and sometimes 11 times a day. He tries to get in to see his doctor for a check-up every 90 days. He runs, bikes, trains with weights, and plays sports.

"I'm trying to live with the disease in the best way I can," he says. "And I've never felt better in my life."

He says he has more energy since he's been on tight control, though he's had more insulin reactions, too. He figures that goes with the territory. "If you've had diabetes for 15 or 20 years, you're going to have reactions, every possible place you can have one." The reason is hypoglycemia unawareness—he doesn't get the early warning signs of a reaction. Before he knows it, his thinking is impaired.

"You know the first thing most people who are having an insulin reaction say? 'Oh, I'm fine. There's nothing at all wrong with me. I don't need anything.'

"I have to be really aware of that, and that's the reason I check my blood as often as I do. I'm onstage a lot, and I have to make sure I'm making the right decisions at the right time for the right reasons. I don't want to be making those decisions when I'm out there in never-never land.

"Clark Rose and the guys in my band, many of whom I've been with for 10 years, keep an eye on me. That's something I do need."

Still, he thinks tight control is worth it. "I want to live longer," he says. "I do believe we are living in an age when we'll find a cure, and I want to be here when it happens."

Collie is doing his bit to hurry that cure along. The Mark Collie Celebrity Race for Diabetes Cure premiered last October. With racing legend Richard Petty as Grand Marshall, professional race car drivers competed alongside country music stars, some of whom were racing for the first time.

"The event raised only $180,000," Collie says. "But we hope to raise $400,000 next year. We've already got 40 country music stars signed for next year."

The first year's proceeds established the Mark Collie Foundation. The foundation made a donation to the ADA Tennessee Affiliate. Another grant went to Vanderbilt University, in Nashville, in the name of Larrie Londin, a popular Nashville sessions musician who died from diabetes-related complications.

Collie plans to fund fellowships for new researchers, to get them interested in diabetes as a career. "We want to attract good researchers before they go into other areas," he says.

"Research dollars are becoming harder to get. So many people have the misconception that the disease is curable, or at least controllable. I'm of the opinion that it's not even controllable. We can treat it, but if we could control it, it wouldn't kill you or take your kidneys or your eyesight.

"It's come down to individuals who are committed and will raise the money. I hope we can generate millions of dollars in the next few years."

Staying Power

But Collie's not abandoning music for fundraising. His latest album, *Tennessee Plates,* is due out in July. He's out on the road doing concerts 8 months of the year, and he writes and records the other 4 months.

"I don't know if there's a correct way to write songs," he says. "I just try to write down some thoughts every day, and some days I get lucky.

"I try to collaborate with the hit makers here in town who don't record, but who have ideas that need to be heard. They'll maybe spark an idea within me, and maybe together we can collaborate to make a better song. John Lennon and Paul McCartney wrote wonderful songs independent of one another, but I think there's no question that their collaborations were the strongest.

"For me, the most important thing is to leave a few songs that will last and will communicate to people years from now. I just want to create music that will take country music into the next millennium. The names, the faces, the stars change. The only thing that lasts is the music."

Marie McCarren is associate editor of Diabetes Forecast.

Arnold Chase: Wizard of Ahhhs

by *Marcia Levine Mazur*

This article appeared in *Diabetes Forecast,* October 1996.

Sure, Arnold Chase of Hartford, Connecticut, is a genius. But he's not your run-of-the-mill Einstein.

Although he taught himself electronics in the second grade, started one of the most powerful TV stations in the country in his 20s, and reads 100 newspapers and journals a month, Chase has a bit of the devil in him, too. He loves to scare people.

Just join the thousands who tremble their way through the electronic scare-a-thon he created, helped finance, and to a great extent, built. It's called Haunted Happenings, and it lies in wait from October 1 through 31 in the basement—40,000 square feet—of the old G. Fox Department Store in downtown Hartford, Connecticut.

It was Chase who dreamed up this electronic nightmare, and it was he who wired it into life.

And while Chase could easily hire others to do the grunt work, he's a hands-on kind of wizard who stays involved in every phase of Haunted Happenings, from the first blueprint to the last hammer stroke.

He doesn't do just the glitzy stuff, either. You can find him with the regular workmen—installing sets, arranging displays, tinkering, testing, and trying new ideas until the second before the doors open.

Some of the milder horrors he's created: "spiders" dropping from the ceiling; electricity crackling fiendishly through Dr. Frankenstein's laboratory; severed, but still-talking heads served on a platter; a mine shaft gripped in the throes of an earthquake; and elevators that wrench themselves off course. (Chase managed that feat by installing real elevators—salvaged from another building—and rigging them to jerk sideways unexpectedly.)

No wonder Haunted Happenings is not for children under 8, or that Chase gets such pleasure standing in the midst of the mayhem, reveling in every goose bump his house of horror raises.

Mystery

What makes a pillar of the community, successful entrepreneur, and electronic genius—even one with a world-class sense of humor—donate thousands of dollars and uncounted hours to such an extravaganza? Diabetes.

He, and two of his four children, 16-year-old William and 8-year-old Melissa, have type 1 diabetes (14-year-old Sara and 9-year-old Allison do not have the disease).

Chase donates all of the profits from Haunted Happenings to the ADA Connecticut Affiliate, with whom he has maintained a long-term relationship. He is a current member of the affiliate's Board of Directors.

Prancing Reindeer

But wait. There's a gentler side to Arnold Chase, and it surfaces in November. That's when he buries Haunted Happenings—well, seals it up—and breathes life into a downright sweetheart of a fund-raiser: Winter Wonderland.

This time he personally animates six floors of electronic marvels, but now there's a singing forest of the nations (some trees are 12 feet tall), herds of prancing reindeer, and a child-size Santa's village with the old gentleman himself in attendance. He even displays a collection of magnificent doll houses as well as antique and Shirley Temple dolls.

This is the fourth year for Haunted Happenings, the third for Winter Wonderland, and both are howling successes. Visitors line up for hours, and tour buses, filled to capacity, roll in from a 100-mile radius. In 1995 alone the two combined brought in more than $100,000 to the American Diabetes Association.

Both events also bring thousands of holiday shoppers back to downtown Hartford.

Tryout

Where did this love of magic, this sense of wonder, come from? "I was born with an innate curiosity," Chase explains. "I love to see how things work."

That led Chase to a surprising experiment when he was in his early teens—testing his urine for sugar. "It seems funny now," he says. "As far as we knew, no one in the family had diabetes, but I just love to try things."

The test was negative, but the teenager recognized the symptoms of the disease when they did appear the week before his 16th birthday.

"Of course," he adds, "I wasn't thrilled with the prospect of having diabetes, but I was fascinated by the equipment. Besides, I thought diabetes presented an intriguing challenge. I wanted to see how good I could become at controlling it."

Starting Early

Chase's scientific bent surfaced early. He taught himself electronics in the second grade, built TV antennas when he was 11, and won a state science fair award for making a Doppler-shift radar system at 14.

While still in his teens, Chase wired a home intercom system; built several color TV sets; repaired his school's phonographs, movie projectors, and P.A. system; and delved into short-wave radio.

His boundless curiosity led him to experiment with photography, ham radio, and magic; he mastered them all. Young Arnold far preferred rewiring a TV set to playing ball.

At 16, Chase became aware of an FCC-approved, but unused, TV channel—a great rarity—and tucked the knowledge away for 12 years. When he finally applied for ownership, prominent people—Gene Autry was one—competed with him for it. Chase hung on for four more years and finally won a legal battle for the station.

Then he sat down at his work bench and helped build the transmitter that put his own TV station, Channel 61, on the air. "At one time, it had the most powerful signal in the country," he adds.

At 27, he began gathering the world's largest collection of antique television sets, even figuring out how to rebuild junked sets that only he recognized as rare and valuable. It was Chase who rescued the original RCA TV that introduced the country to television at New York's 1939 World's Fair.

The antique TV collection became so historically important it was put on display at the Smithsonian Institution in Washington, D.C. (Now sold, it is part of the permanent collection of the MZTV Museum in Toronto, Canada.)

Today, Arnold Chase, a successful businessman, still carries his repair kit for electronic equipment in his pocket.

Though he could easily coast through life, Chase has been known to tumble out of bed on a stormy night and service the radar equipment that feeds his own New England Weather Service.

Actually, he loves tinkering with any kind of equipment, especially that belonging to the Weather Service. "And I love to track storms around the country," he adds.

What To Do?

Before there was a TV station and the New England Weather Service, before there was his Chase Communications and Communications Site Management, even before there were stop-your-heart fund-raisers, 18-year-old Arnold Chase had the same problem most high school seniors have: What to take in college?

Should he pursue electronics, telecommunications, or American history? With his near-limitless areas of interest, choosing a college major was a tough call.

So Chase entered a business school, Babson College in Wellesley, Massachusetts, on the theory that a knowledge of business would help him profit from his other interests.

At school, his churning mind glommed onto everything, even if it wasn't in a textbook. Chase displayed an uncanny ability to diagnose and repair auto engines—as well as pinball machines.

But he had a rude awakening in his first postgraduate venture—he and some friends attempted a real estate deal. It didn't pan out.

So when his father, David, president of Chase Enterprises, a real-estate-oriented company, bought Hartford's Radio Station WTIC AM and FM in 1974, Chase moved into telecommunications.

And A Little Romance?

While Arnold was arranging his professional future, a friend insisted on arranging a blind date for him. "You'd be good for each other," the friend told Chase.

"I turned his offer down several times before I ran out of excuses and was trapped into going," Chase recalls.

The date was with an art teacher named Sandra Dakers. The friend was right; they were a good match. The couple was married 1 year later.

The Best And Worst Of Times

By 1984, Arnold and Sandra were raising two children and living happily ever after. Yet Chase recalls 1984 as both "the best and the worst year of my life."

It was the best year because it was the summer of 1984 when Chase realized a life-long dream—establishing his own TV station.

And it was the worst year because, a few weeks before the station went on the air, Chase noticed that their oldest child, 4-year-old William, was inexplicably wetting himself. When Chase tested his son, he realized that William had diabetes.

About the same time, doctors discovered that Sandra had breast cancer. William's diabetes was brought under control; and Sandra was operated on successfully.

Then, 5 years later, in the spring of 1989, Chase noticed that 17-month-old Melissa was soaking through her diapers. "Something told me to test her, too," he recalls. Her blood sugar was close to 200.

Sandra found it difficult to accept the fact that two of her children now had diabetes. "When William was diagnosed, we were heartbroken," she says, "but when our youngest, a little girl only 17 months old, developed it, that hit me really hard."

Lightening Up

Things have lightened considerably since then. "We caught the children's diabetes early, and it's been 12 years since my wife's surgery, and, happily, she is just fine," Chase says.

He has imparted his "you can handle this" attitude to his children. Like their father, William and Melissa eat well and test their blood glucose a minimum of six times a day.

"Even though monitoring is easy, most people don't test anywhere near the amount they should," Chase says. "Regular monitoring is critical to the successful management of diabetes."

The regimen works well for the three Chases. "After my last exam, my eye doctor said that even after 29 years of diabetes there is no way of knowing from my eyes that I have the disease," Arnold says. "And the children's HbA_{1c} tests show them in the almost nondiabetic range."

Sandra helps keep the children's diabetes regimen on target. "I do things like taking field trips with them," she says. The other two children, Sara and Allison, are also very supportive.

The Chases also talk to parents of other newly diagnosed children.

Sowing The Seed

It was Sandra who unwittingly sowed the seed for Haunted Happenings.

She hoped to entice William and Melissa into staying home rather than trick-or-treating for candy on Halloween. So she put up a few modest decorations outside of the house.

Arnold gravitated toward the project like electricity to a lightning rod. "I love electronics and mechanical things," he says, "and this was a great chance to play with them."

Soon the Chase home displayed flashing lights, a mail box that opened and slammed shut by itself ("You should have seen the mailman the first time that happened!" Chase recalls), figures cavorting on the lawn, and a witch holding her own bloodied head over a caldron. Visitors had to make it through a 60-foot canvas-covered "tunnel of terror" to reach the front door.

For 10 years the family—and most of Hartford—loved it. Gobs of gaping visitors filled the street each October.

Then Arnold and Sandra visited a haunted house that did more than entertain. It raised money for charity, and another light flashed—this time in Arnold's mind.

Why not make his Halloween creation a fund-raiser for diabetes?

It took years of planning, starting with a search for the right site. There were a few stops along the way. The first Haunted Happenings was held in an abandoned roller rink. ("Even though the rink was half the size of our present location, that first Haunted Happenings attracted more than 11,000 people," Chase adds.)

A Special Legacy

Arnold Chase's upbeat attitude and generous public spirit reflect those of his parents, Rhoda and David.

David Chase, born David Ciesla near Warsaw, Poland, was imprisoned in Auschwitz, the infamous Nazi death camp, when he was 14. He was 16 when the war ended and liberation came.

David made it to America, where he was aided by the Jewish community of Hartford. He learned English, attended school, founded Chase Enterprises, and built it into a real estate and communications empire.

Today David is president of Chase Enterprises and Arnold is executive vice president. The elder Chases' remaining child, Cheryl, is general counsel and executive vice president.

Forbes magazine has listed David as one of the most successful businessmen in America. But he has not attempted to erase his past; David still displays the blue numbers tattooed on his arm at Auschwitz.

A few years ago David, a confidant of world leaders, took up a suggestion made to him by Pope John Paul II to help Poland modernize.

Now Chase Enterprises is doing just that. It has sold its eight radio and five TV stations in the United States (although it still has many other holdings) and has become the largest cable TV provider in Poland. There are plans to expand into other businesses there as well.

But the rink wasn't the answer, and, with help from the ADA Connecticut Affiliate and the City of Hartford, Chase finally nailed down a perfect locale twice its size—the basement of the empty downtown G. Fox Department Store.

Once he stepped inside, Chase never looked back. He immediately set the second Haunted Happenings into production (attendance more than doubled), and created Winter Wonderland. Haunted Happenings still works its October magic in the basement of the building, while Winter Wonderland charms November visitors on the six upper floors.

Chase continues to ratchet up the fear and enchantment of his electronic wonders and each year more people respond to both of them. "We sold a total of 37,000 tickets in 1995 and we're aiming for 50,000 this year."

"Arnold put himself on the line for these fund-raisers," Sandra says. "They were his idea and his work. If these projects had failed, he'd have had to take the blame." But there was probably little chance of failure. Arnold Chase is a born winner.

And a man forever young.

Marcia Levine Mazur is senior editor of Diabetes Forecast.

Kenneth Padilla: For His People

by Marcia Levine Mazur

This article appeared in *Diabetes Forecast,* January 1994.

Despite spectacular desert vistas and the nearness of the mighty Rio Grande, life in New Mexico's San Felipe Indian Pueblo can be grim, especially when your family has been devastated by diabetes.

Kenneth Padilla, a 38-year-old San Felipe Indian, knows all about it.

Although his father, Pablo, has no known diabetes in his family, his mother, Marcella, has more than enough in hers.

Marcella developed type 2 diabetes when Padilla was a boy. Her two brothers also had the disease. Because they received only the most basic level of care, both brothers eventually required leg amputations, and both died young from further complications caused by diabetes.

Padilla's own older brother, Joseph, also was diagnosed when Padilla was a boy. He, too, developed complications he could not handle, and died in his 30s.

Padilla's mother lost a leg to diabetic complications, but she has responded to newer techniques, and is in good health today.

In 1986, at age 32, Padilla heard the same diagnosis: type 2 diabetes. He has dropped about 40 pounds since then, and keeps in shape by watching his diet, walking whenever possible, and running several times a week.

Fighting Back

Although diabetes is rife throughout the Pueblo, the San Felipe Indians are fighting back. Change and hope are in the air and Kenneth Padilla exemplifies both.

Born in a two-room adobe home, he lived his early years among eight members of his extended family. There was no phone, plumbing, or electricity. The family got its light from a kerosene lamp and heat from a wood stove and a fireplace. To get to nearby Albuquerque, they had to ask one of the Pueblo's three or four car owners for a lift.

With unemployment high in the Pueblo, Padilla went to Albuquerque to earn a nursing assistant's degree, then took several jobs in his field there before joining the Pueblo's health program.

Today, Padilla, his mother and father, his girlfriend, and their four children—who were born in a hospital—live in a three-bedroom house with a kitchen, living room, and bathroom. They are warmed by a gas heater, enjoy movies on their VCR, phone conversations with friends, football on TV, and trips to town in their own pickup truck.

In 1991, Padilla became one of four Community Health Representatives (CHR) working for the Pueblo of San Felipe. The San Felipe Tribe, through the authority of Public Law 93-638, contracted from the U.S. Indian Health Service to provide medical services to the Pueblo. Padilla works in the CHR office located in the Pueblo.

His job: to help educate his fellow Indians on the prevention and treatment of type 2 diabetes. But for Padilla, diabetes education reaches far beyond a job description.

Always Available

The soft-spoken Padilla is always available to see that a Pueblo resident gets to a medical appointment, or that an Indian with little English understands the doctor's instructions.

He visits the homes of Pueblo residents who have diabetes, explaining the importance of self-health care and advising them when to go to the doctor.

Padilla speaks to the children in the reservation school, stressing the need to stay close to a normal weight and eat well. "It's particularly important to talk to the kids," he says.

Padilla adds, "The good thing about type 2 diabetes in the Pueblo is that at least we don't see children with diabetes." (Type 2 diabetes, the kind prevalent among Native

Americans, hardly ever occurs in children. Children who get diabetes in childhood are far more likely to have type 1 diabetes, which is rare among Native Americans.)

Because the Pueblo's next generation is so important to Padilla, he has just finished coordinating a diabetes workshop as well as a presentation on diabetes prevention for parents. He is now preparing for an upcoming elementary school health fair.

"We're also organizing fundraising events because we want to get a wellness center with an exercise area for the Pueblo," he adds.

His supervisor, Mike Paseno, sums up Kenneth Padilla this way: "He is very unselfish, very concerned with the well-being of the health of people in the Pueblo, especially people afflicted with diabetes."

But Padilla's work isn't easy; it's always difficult to convince people to change their lifestyles. "Many people have trouble accepting the fact that they have diabetes, especially the elderly, but they are learning."

Pueblo Life

The San Felipe Pueblo, where Padilla lives and works, is a village of about 3,000. "I know just about everyone there except the small children," he says. It is one of 19 pueblos in New Mexico and, like each of them, has its own feast days and traditions. It also has its own language, known as Keres.

The language isn't easy, with many meanings for one word, but its use today demonstrates the Pueblo's interest in its own culture. Older residents speak mainly Keres; the middle generation speaks both Keres and English; and the children are taught to speak both Keres and English.

Padilla explains the ins and outs of choosing which language to speak. "If my youngest sister comes with her husband, who is from another tribe, or my second oldest sister visits with her husband, who is Caucasian, we speak English, because they don't understand Keres. But we speak Keres at night when we eat dinner, then stick to English again especially when there is a football game on TV."

The Pueblo itself is also changing. Once almost all homes were adobe, a kind of brick made primarily of mud and straw hardened by the heat of the sun. Today, you can also see houses made of cement block and timber. A few trailers dot the land.

Because many Native Americans live together in extended families, many elderly parents share living space with their children and grandchildren, which greatly enhances the contact among the generations.

To Your Health

Health standards have also risen in the San Felipe Pueblo. The message health workers such as Padilla carry is paying off. And thanks mainly to Padilla himself, many of his people are now aware of diabetes, its prevention, and treatment.

Still, he knows it's an uphill battle to get people to adopt a healthy diet with all the food choices that are out there today. "I never had a soft drink when I was a kid," he says, "but when I'm driving to work in the morning, I see kids waiting for the buses eating chips and drinking soft drinks."

His own family represents a middle ground. His mother still prepares a kind of wild spinach that grows in nearby fields, has given up using lard, and prepares fresh vegetable casseroles from her husband's garden. But she also buys more foods than ever from the supermarket.

"Even though we are more aware of a good diet, we can't really go back to our old ways," Padilla explains. "For instance, my dad loves to garden, and he owned 75 apple trees and I-don't-know-how-many peach trees. But they stopped bearing fruit and he cut them down. Now we buy apples and peaches from the store."

The staple of the Pueblo, however, has long been tortillas. "The tortillas are round and flat like pita bread, but you put nothing into them," Inez Lucero, a colleague of Padilla's, explains. But she isn't sure how they came to be an Indian food. "History books say the Spaniards taught us how to make them, but the corn and wheat for the flour came from the Indians. So it isn't clear."

What is clear is that the tortillas are so popular that most Pueblo Indians choose to cook on wood-burning stoves because it is easy to make tortillas on them.

Lasting Traditions

Although Padilla is pleased with the recent advances in health care, he bemoans some of the Pueblo's cultural losses. "We used to visit each other's families, going from house to house. And people would come in, and hug each other. Today people are afraid to touch. They don't hug anymore."

Padilla adds, "I hope our traditions last, and that our children continue talking our language. Mainly I hope that a cure can be found for diabetes. That is why we are doing all this. But we are really just starting. There are more plans under way."

Although life may be easier in cities such as Albuquerque, Kenneth Padilla is happy to be among his own people. "I would rather live here on the Pueblo," he says.

Marcia Levine Mazur is senior editor of Diabetes Forecast.

George Thompson: Seeking the Sublime

by Marie McCarren

This article appeared in *Diabetes Forecast,* November 1996.

George Thompson can almost hear the thoughts behind the stares. "People think, 'Aw, poor bastard, he's blind,' and I think, poor bastard indeed, poor bastard, he's diabetic! If he gets away from his insulin, he's in trouble; if he takes too much of it, he's going to have a reaction.

"I'd be blind 10 times over compared to the big D. That's the scary one. It's a wolf at your heels, and if you ignore it, it will sink its teeth into your calf. It could blow at any seam. The kinds of things that can happen to you—to your feet, to your kidneys—serious stuff."

Thompson is speaking with a new heat that you might not expect from someone who's had diabetes for 38 years. But diabetes has a way of stoking anger. For Thompson that came last year, when his doctor told him there was a small amount of protein in his urine. In 10 years, Thompson may be looking at kidney failure.

"It's making me sore," says Thompson, 50, a high school counselor and part-time musician in Portland, Oregon. "I've had a very good life, and if I died tomorrow, I'd have no regrets. I'm not afraid of seeing the end of things. I just don't want it to be a dismal, bleak, and dreadful end that pulls down my family and friends. That would make me very angry."

Then the flame dies back.

"Every once in a while, I get a little cross with the Almighty. But when I consider the breaks I've been given, the discoveries I've made, and—this may sound a little highblown—when I consider how incredibly blessed I've been, then to complain about the things I've been offered as a challenge is like a little kid losing his temper because he's gotten himself coiled up in his blankets."

Don't Worry?

When Thompson was diagnosed with diabetes at age 12, he already thought of diabetes as a "black cloud." His sister Kitty, 12 years his senior, had had diabetes since she was 13. She had the inevitable conflicts with her parents over all the time-consuming must-do's of that era's diabetes regimens.

When Thompson was diagnosed, his parents tried a new tack. "They did me the greatest favor by leaving it up to me. Any kind of intrusion would have made matters worse."

Though Thompson appreciated his parents' hands-off approach, he says the doctors should have given him more of the harsh facts.

"We were told as kids: Don't worry about it. You'll live a normal life. They should have said, 'You have something that can really get you. You have to live carefully. Diabetes is no joke.'"

But then Thompson admits, almost in the same breath, that maybe he wouldn't have listened.

"I was told by a terrible nurse practitioner, a horrible old battle-ax, 'You have to weigh your food every day.' Weigh my food? I'm a teenager! I tried. I really tried. That lasted about 2 weeks.

"I'm not blaming anybody. People did the best they could. Perhaps if the doctors had laid it on a little heavy, I would have recoiled. I don't know."

One-Barn School

For whatever reason, Thompson rolled through his teens and 20s not paying much mind to diabetes management.

"My control as a teenager was what you would expect any teenager's to be who wasn't athletic," he says. "If I were as athletic then as I am now—God! I've so often thought about this. I'd rewind the cameras and take my fifteenth year over again and this time run every morning, and this time not smoke because it's cool, and this time not get drunk with my buddies. It's just ridiculous to do those things if you're a diabetic, but teenagers do some pretty stupid things." In high school, Thompson did test his urine for glucose, but after high school, he quit testing completely.

Though his diabetes management plan lacked direction, Thompson's career path didn't. While at Middlesex, a prep school in Concord, Massachusetts, he discovered his calling: to be a teacher.

Thompson studied history in undergraduate and graduate school. After teaching for a year at his old prep school, Thompson, his wife, Margot, and baby daughter, Lise, went back to Thompson's home state of Oregon while he finished his master's thesis. And there the Thompsons got a harebrained idea: They would open a school.

"It was the '70s," Thompson explains. "We were idealistic."

With money he had inherited from his grandfather, Thompson bought some land and an old barn in Neskowin, Oregon. For a year, he went stumping at churches and granges. He told people that this school would be different—a throw-back to the one-room schoolhouse. A family environment. A place where kids would have a sense of community.

Parents—from city workers to loggers—went for the idea. In the fall of 1973, Neskowin Valley School opened with 20 students aged 3 to 6. George Thompson was headmaster and one-half of the teaching staff.

Red Curtain

The winter after the school opened, Thompson started having trouble with one of his eyes. Thompson's doctor told him about laser photocoagulation, which at that time was an experimental treatment for retinopathy. The doctor warned Thompson that laser treatment might cause some loss of peripheral vision.

What Thompson took from that conversation was that laser treatment might not do any good but it would definitely do harm. He decided against laser treatments, a reasonable decision at the time. (Today, laser photocoagulation is the treatment of choice for proliferative retinopathy. When retinopathy is advanced and requires extensive laser treatment, there may be some loss of peripheral vision, but this is minor compared with the amount of vision that is saved.)

Throughout the spring, Thompson's eyes got worse. In July, doctors put him in the hospital on Valium, in the hopes that with bed rest, his eyes would stop bleeding. While he was in the hospital, Margot was admitted to the same hospital in labor with their second baby. The Thompsons had studied Lamaze, so Thompson joined his wife. After a day of difficult labor, Geordie was born. And within a week, a red curtain had dropped over Thompson's eyes.

That September, Neskowin Valley School opened for its second year with 30 students and three teachers. From home, while coping with his vision loss, Thompson tried to uphold his duties as headmaster.

In January, Thompson went to St. Louis, Mo., for a vitrectomy from a renowned surgeon. But Thompson's retinas were beyond help. The 6-hour surgery didn't restore any of his vision, and it left him with a lot of pain. In February and March, surgeons tried to relieve the pressure in his right eye. Finally, they removed the eye.

"The relief was so incredible that I couldn't even grieve over the lost eye," says Thompson.

Now with no hope of regaining any vision, Thompson enrolled at the Oregon Rehabilitation Center for the Blind, in Salem, where he lived for 2 months, learning skills such as reading Braille.

When Neskowin Valley School opened for its third year, again with more students, Thompson was back as teacher, headmaster, and chief fundraiser. And it seemed he had adjusted extraordinarily well to being blind.

"I was angry, but I didn't know it," Thompson says. "I was too busy being this phoenix. I tried to get people to believe along with me that my blindness was nothing. I was a guy who had overcome blindness.

"But you can only do that for a while. It becomes tiresome. You have to eventually accept your blindness, and then you are just blind."

Student And Counselor

Meanwhile, the school continued to grow, and Thompson continued as headmaster and teacher. Thirteen years after it opened, enrollment was up to 85 and the staff was up to 12.

By then Thompson was ready to give up the long hours of a headmaster. He turned over the title to the property to the school's nonprofit corporation. (Neskowin Valley School is still in operation today, with about 90 students.)

Thompson worked for a year as director of a rehab center for people with vision impairments, then got back to teaching. He joined the staff at Catlin-Gabel, an independent school in Portland, as the eighth-grade English teacher.

Last year, Thompson started a new career, as high school counselor at Catlin-Gabel. He has had some unofficial experience. When the school was without a counselor, kids often went to Thompson with their problems. But Thompson knew he needed more than that. As soon as he took the position, Thompson started taking classes in counseling at Lewis and Clark College in Portland.

"The great thing about taking a class in an on-the-job training situation like this is that you soak up everything. You want to know everything that the professor is telling you."

But learning as he goes, Thompson worries about all he hasn't learned yet. He studies on the weekends and calls on other counselors for advice.

"When you're a counselor, you're supposed to be in the know," he says. "I'm using my intuition, stretching it as far as I can, and shooting from the hip a lot."

He might harbor some doubts about his current abilities, but students who have known him don't. Rachel Cohen, 24, who now works at a nonprofit organization in New York City, graduated from Catlin-Gabel. She met Thompson when he subbed in the high school and now counts him as a friend.

"George has a holistic method of teaching," says Cohen. "He gets the kids engaged by integrating poetry and art into the lesson. He introduces kids to life.

"Knowing how he was as a teacher, I can only imagine the creative and innovative ways he will bring to his counseling."

Cohen says Thompson is unlike many adults in that he actually listens to teens without ever being patronizing or condescending. She also thinks his blindness helps kids relate to him.

"Adolescents—especially young women—often have bad feelings about body image," says Cohen. "Kids feel loved by him, not despite their appearances but without regard to their appearances.

"He's magnetic. He's always surrounded by a cloud of young people. You'll see a pack of seventh graders helping him down the stairs. But it's not charity that people feel for George. He commands respect because he gives it. He listens to people and doesn't prejudge them."

Music In The Mayhem

While he's launching his new day job, Thompson's other career—as a musician—is reaching comfortable maturity. Thompson and teachers Tom Tucker and Craig Stewart make up the folk group Sligo Ross. Thompson may never be able to quit his day job, but he's been having a grand time as part of Sligo Ross for 16 years. Thompson sings, and plays guitar and mandola. Sligo Ross performs mainly original music, written by Thompson or Stewart.

"It keeps us fresh," says Thompson. "Warming up old covers—that doesn't interest me. I'm too old for that."

Last year, Sligo Ross cut its first CD and played a 14-day summer concert tour in New England. Back home, they prefer to play house concerts: 20 to 40 people gathered in a private home, which Thompson says is the best way to hear Sligo Ross' unmiked instruments.

The worst way to hear their music is as background to an event. The instruments and close harmonies of the singers get lost in the chaos.

"One night we played for a convention of contractors," Thompson recalls. "They had gotten into the alcohol, and they were bellowing and raging and laughing and hooting. We were standing right next to each other, and we couldn't hear where we were in the song. We got $500, and it was the most thankless $500 we earned. It did help us cut our CD, but geez!"

Sligo Ross has decided to forgo the big bucks and keep writing songs with the expectation that people will actually listen to the words. Thompson recently wrote a song about what he sees, called "Night Sky."

"When moments that are sublime or tranquil or beautiful happen, the insides of my eyes light up like a summer sky. When I'm troubled or perplexed or distracted or fearful, everything's a dull gray.

"I've written several poems about it, but this is the first time I've ever written a song about it. And you know what? It's a good song. It works. I've got some interesting chord sequences in there, and the words really express what I'm trying to say.

"We were practicing it the other night, and the other two boys started getting into it. Boy, it started to cook. There's a feeling you get when your song begins to strike up a life of its own, when it starts to become itself. It steps away from your ownership of it, and then the song has its own personality. That's a really nice moment."

Larger Truth

"One takes a hit by a two-by-four in a variety of ways in one's life, and blindness happened to be mine," Thompson says. "Sometimes, we're pretty clueless. And then something comes along—and it's funny how adversity does this—and it forces you to shuffle your cards a little bit, and you see that life is very much worth living.

"I could repeat all the fatuous aphorisms I heard from other people when I went blind: 'You'll see in different ways.' 'It will build character.' All that claptrap. But blindness squared my sails. I would not trade who I am today, with blindness, for who I was then. I know that sounds bloody convenient."

Thompson has less-kind things to say about diabetes and impending kidney disease, but he's dealing with those, too. In recent years, he's gotten more serious about his health.

He tries to keep his blood glucose levels as controlled as possible, but he is plagued by insulin reactions. He doesn't get the early warnings he used to, and the aftermath lasts hours. "It's like being hungover," he says. However, he recently took a 4-day canoe trip and was delighted to make it through with no reactions.

He exercises every day—either with a good, hard walk or a workout on his cross-country ski machine. ("You don't feel quite so like a gerbil in a cage.") He quit drinking and smoking 10 years ago. He takes an ACE inhibitor, a drug that may slow the progression of his kidney disease.

"My doctor said that in 10 years I'll have to be thinking about the possibility of dialysis. That gives me until I'm 60, and if I take really good care of myself in those 10 years, maybe it'll be another 10 years."

Thompson finds strength in music, meditation, exercise, and his faith in God. "Having a faith," he says, "one suspects there is a larger truth."

He says that if one had to put a name to his "religion," it might be Buddhism, Sufism, Hindu Mysticism, or St. Francis Mysticism.

"I grew up in the church," Thompson says, "but I had to throw all that out before the real McCoy made itself felt in my life. All the institutional rigidities don't interest me in the slightest. I don't think churches are where we find God.

"I tossed Him aside my freshman year of college; He came back with a rush when I was 23. My daughter was sick, and I asked Him to help me out. Having not talked to Him for 5 or 6 years, it was 'Hey mister, remember me?'

"Then it was a series of slow steps, culminating 3 or 4 years after my blindness."

But please don't call him "saved."

"Being saved makes it sound like I was condemned before," he says. "The only condemnation was my ignorance. I woke up, or somebody woke me up."

And when the character-building aspects of diabetes and kidney disease elude him, Thompson looks to the larger truth and concentrates on how he has been blessed.

"I've been given a blessing of a fairly strong intuition, which is why I'm a counselor.

"I love children, and their company and companionship are a blessing.

"I have a wonderful family. My wife and I have been together for 29 years, and I have two fabulous kids.

"I have a happy nature."

Marie McCarren is associate editor of Diabetes Forecast.

Andrea Carroll: Mission to the Ukraine

by Marcia Levine Mazur

This article appeared in *Diabetes Forecast,* September 1994.

"It was the children," says Andrea (Andy) Carroll of Windsor, California. "I just could not forget the children."

Carroll is talking about the eight girls and boys with diabetes she met in a Ukrainian hospital in 1990.

"I'm a registered dietitian and a certified diabetes educator, but I'd never seen anything like it. They were in ketoacidosis, the last stage of diabetes. Their eyes were sunken and they were emaciated—you could see their bones beneath their skin, smell the tell-tale fruity smell on their breath.

"Those children were very sick, every single one of them, and there I was, an American who'd had the same disease for more than 20 years, but I was in perfect health. They couldn't believe it. They were blown away."

So was Carroll. "I sat right down with an interpreter and told them about things they'd never known, blood glucose testing, good nutrition, and daily multiple insulin injections. Then I left some syringes and insulin, and gave one young girl, Natasha, my meter and test strips and told her, 'When you run out of these, let me know.'"

But Carroll did more: She launched a program that now spans continents, fills cross-country trucks and international flights with diabetes supplies, and dispenses millions of dollars worth of educational and medical goods in Ukraine, part of the former Soviet Union.

Curious Remark

Although it now seems that Andrea Carroll was destined to meet those eight Ukrainian children, it was only a travel agent's offhand remark that brought her to them.

She'd heard the comment 9 months earlier while arranging a European vacation that would culminate in a tour of Ukraine from a boat on the Dnieper River.

The European jaunt was hers to plan; the boat segment was under the auspices of a nonprofit educational organization called Promoting Enduring Peace.

But no extended hospital visit was on the agenda until a travel agent remarked, "When you're in Ukraine, don't tip with money. Tip with gifts. You know, lipstick, pantyhose, syringes."

"Syringes?" Carroll was stunned. She knew all about syringes. She'd had type 1 diabetes for 23 years. "Why syringes?"

The agent had heard that children with diabetes in the former Soviet Union had only limited quantities of diabetes supplies.

That was enough for Carroll. She bought and begged 1,000 syringes, purchased other diabetes supplies, then dragged everything around Europe with her until she could load them onto the plane to Kiev.

There she hooked up with the Dnieper River tour and asked a Ukrainian doctor where she might deliver her supplies. The doctor brought Carroll to the hospital in Kiev. And there she met the eight children.

Letter From Natasha

As soon as Carroll saw how diabetes had devastated the children's health, she promised herself she'd do more than leave medical goods behind. But even after she returned to the United States, Carroll wasn't sure how she could fulfill that promise until a letter from little Natasha brought it all into focus.

Natasha was the girl to whom Carroll had given the meter and test strips. Although her letter was in Ukrainian, the accompanying picture spoke for itself. There was Natasha holding the empty strip box upside down; she had run out.

Carroll forwarded a copy to the test strip manufacturer, who sent back a case of strips and two more meters.

"When I saw how eager people were to help," she recalls, "I knew I could do more, much more." And the idea for the Ukrainian Diabetes Project was born.

Why?

Why should Andrea Carroll devote herself to helping children with diabetes thousands of miles away?

Part of the answer is the affinity she feels with the people of Ukraine, the land her family emigrated from nearly a century ago. She knows that in America she has always had easy access to diabetes care. She's lived an active life and is an avid bicyclist and backpacker. "My disease has made few incursions into my lifestyle," she says, "but how different that would be if I had grown up in Ukraine."

Then, too, Carroll has a special concern for children, perhaps stemming from her own happy childhood as one of 13 youngsters in a closeknit Chicago family.

And she also knows what it's like to have insulin-dependent diabetes; she was diagnosed at 14.

But there's an even more compelling reason.

Holding a vial of insulin, Carroll says simply, "I can take this insulin for granted. It gives me life while children in Ukraine are dying for lack of it. To them diabetes is a horrible disease that makes them sick, stunts their growth, and kills them. And all because they don't have something I can buy at any corner drugstore. As a person with diabetes, I couldn't walk away from that."

Like almost all medical equipment, insulin is extremely hard to come by in Ukraine, with few syringes and absolutely no blood glucose testing meters or strips. "Diabetes treatment there is about where it was in the United States in the '20s or '30s," Carroll says. "They have a system of socialized medicine, but it's useless without the medicine."

Still, Carroll feels Ukrainian children are blessed. "With all their troubles, these are the most caring, gentle people I have ever seen."

And So It Began

Carroll began her project by asking for donations from her family and friends with diabetes. "I don't remember who I called," she says, laughing. "I know I contacted pharmacies and local sales reps. Everyone was extremely helpful. The diabetic supply manufacturers particularly have been incredibly generous. They have given so many supplies. I just couldn't have done it without them."

She also listed every donor to the project so the children or their families could write thank-you notes.

But almost immediately Carroll hit barriers more difficult than lack of money and supplies. The first was communications. How could she stay in touch with Kiev when phone calls took days to get through and letters took months, if they arrived at all?

That was solved by an incredible stroke of luck. Santa Rosa, Calif., the city where Carroll worked at the time, is the sister city to a Ukrainian town, Cherkasy, about 80 miles from Kiev.

Because of that, a Santa Rosa citizen had brought a word processor to Cherkasy and set up an electronic mail (e-mail) system. Now Carroll could communicate instantaneously with a Ukrainian city. "It made all the difference," she says. She moved the focus of the project to Cherkasy.

Going Back

Although Carroll had never planned to return to Ukraine, meeting the children changed all that. One year after her first trip, tears filled her eyes as she rushed forward to embrace little Natasha and the others again. But what a difference. Now the children had warm smiles, pink cheeks, and blood glucose levels that approached normal.

Still, they did not yet have their diabetes stabilized. And there were so many more who'd never been reached.

Back in the United States after her second trip, Carroll collected enough supplies to sustain 30 children for 1 year. The following year she established an ongoing diabetes clinic in the city of Cherkasy.

(Carroll explains that two nonprofit, tax-free organizations, Promoting Enduring Peace of Woodmont, Connecticut, and The Diabetic Youth Foundation of Walnut Creek, California, accept checks for the Project without charge. "We take nothing out for administrative costs," she adds.)

But teaching diabetes care in Ukraine brought up another difficulty: the culture gap. "It didn't make sense for me to explain about the monounsaturated fats in olive oil if they couldn't get any olive oil, or to tell children to go swimming if there were no swimming pools," she explains.

Moving In

Carroll realized that there was only one way to learn the culture: Live it. So she arranged to stay with a Ukrainian family for 2 months each year. "That way I could learn what was practical for them," she says.

"But I learned a lot more too. I saw how they survive in the middle of a horrendous economy with unbelievable inflation. In May 1994, it took 40,000 Ukrainian coupons, once called rubles, to equal the value of one American dollar."

She adds, "Everyone there has a garden, not for leisure, but for survival. Even the doctors, who are not well paid, take off at 3 o'clock to work their gardens. Families preserve as much of the produce as they can, and keep extra potatoes, carrots, and beets in cold storage. That's what they live on all winter."

Something else happened, also. As Carroll lived among the Ukrainians, she became enchanted by them. "They are the most generous people I have ever known. They have so few material things, but they give each other—and me—warm, unconditional love."

Carroll is up-front with her employer about her 2-month stays in Ukraine. "When I applied for my job with California's Solano County Nutrition Department of Health and Social Services last January, I told them I had to have 2 months off without pay each summer to go to Ukraine. That was fine with them."

In fact, the department applauds her commitment, and colleagues have contributed to her project. One, Sherry Woodcock, says, "We know what a positive person Andy is. We see how she cares for people in the clinic and we're sure she cares for the people in Ukraine with the same feeling."

Who Will Take These Supplies?

But the very success of the Ukrainian Diabetes Program raised yet another question. How to ship so many goods overseas?

Tracking every lead, Carroll located trucking companies willing to carry goods gratis from California to the East Coast. Still, overseas transport fees took a big chunk out of donated funds. No matter. She put every spare minute she could into collecting goods for the Ukrainian children. It paid off.

This year, her fifth, Carroll had enough diabetes supplies to last 300 children for 1 year and to set up another three clinics in three more Ukrainian towns. But shipping such huge quantities became incredibly costly, until Carroll made a connection with a New Jersey–based private, non-profit organization called Children of Chernobyl Relief Fund. The fund flew 1,800 pounds of Carroll's goods to Ukraine along with their own.

Air Ukraine, the airline Carroll flies on her trips, carried the remaining goods without charge.

Actually, Carroll's shipments contain more than medical supplies. She brings toys, dolls, and stuffed animals donated by Americans who want to help, whether they have diabetes or not. And she brings cartons of the mega-hit that always brings shouts of joy from the Ukrainian youngsters—sugar-free bubblegum.

Carroll also brings with her an assistant who has diabetes. Seeing another healthy person with diabetes reinforces the message that insulin, exercise, good nutrition, and blood glucose monitoring can indeed control this disease, although that still seems like a dream to many Ukrainians.

She also has arranged to have a book on diabetes care translated into Ukrainian by a couple living in California. "They wrote every word of the translation by hand," she adds.

No Ego

Andrea Carroll displays no sense of ego when she talks about her gargantuan mission. "I don't care who gets the credit," she says, "as long as the children get the supplies."

Carroll can see what a great difference the clinics have made. "I remember how horrible it was when we first came. The children were so sick they were emaciated and listless. Certainly, they didn't know anything about their disease, and they and their families expected them to be invalids all their short lives.

"Now I can hardly recognize the same children from one year to the next. They are coming alive. They have a future. They have hope."

Marcia Levine Mazur is senior editor of Diabetes Forecast.

Waking Up With Craig Walker

by Marie McCarren

This article appeared in *Diabetes Forecast,* January 1993.

He's the guy who wakes you up in the morning. Gently. *It's 6:17. And in case you're still half asleep…That's 17 minutes after 6.*

He's the guy who makes you pause while you're brushing your teeth…*Here's the Morning Music Quiz for you: We play a little bit of a song, you tell us the title. We've got some great prizes.*

Craig Walker, 46, has been easing Oregonians into their day for 6 years as the morning radio personality on Portland's K103FM. Although K103 is listed as adult contemporary, his show attracts teenagers as well as their parents, making it one of the top morning shows in the region. What makes more than 100,000 listeners a week choose Walker to be the guy who invades their morning?

"I am their confidant, their friend, their peer," says Walker. "I'm someone they can talk to."

"It's an unusual relationship. I've had a lot of people talk to me about extraordinarily personal things because they think they can. I have people who call me when good things happen in their lives, because I'm someone they wanted to know about their good fortune."

These aren't people who just want to yak on the radio—Walker doesn't have a call-in show. These are people who confide in a guy whose voice they hear on a radio.

Why?

"Some guys will sit on the air and do time and temp. Over the years, I've talked about everything that is going on in my life. When my kids were young, and I was coaching sports teams for them, I'd talk about those things on the air, because the people who were listening were going through the same thing. I talked about the birth of my children, the death of my parents. It really bonds you with your listeners."

He's been on Portland radio for 22 years and is now on his third generation of listeners. And if listeners feel they don't get to know Walker well enough from his radio show, they can watch him on TV every weekday evening. Walker co-anchors *Good Evening,* a news-magazine show. He's the guy in the argyle-knit cardigan, munching on spanakopeta, reminding his fellow Portland residents that the local Greek festival ends this weekend. His co-host, Teresa Richardson, says the charming, witty, warm guy you see on camera is the same one you'll see behind the scenes. "What you see is what you get," she says.

"I try to be myself on both the TV show and the radio," says Walker. "I just talk and laugh. I am one of them, whoever they are."

Walker has recently found another common bond with some of his listeners. A year ago, he was diagnosed with type 1 diabetes. As is his style, he took to the airways with the news, telling his radio listeners the day after he was diagnosed. And just as they'd do for any member of their families, listeners reached out to Walker.

"I was inundated with information about diabetes, and people who called me to tell me about their experiences with diabetes. I found out that I didn't have an inkling about what people were coping with." He did a story on diabetes for *Good Evening,* which was filmed at Walker's home and showed him giving himself a shot of insulin.

"That was just a continuation of the relationship I have with my radio listeners," says Walker. "I hope it really helped the people who have diabetes. I never contemplated that there were people who had it who were having trouble admitting it—they were almost in the closet."

Diabetes educators in the Portland area knew when Walker went public, even without hearing him themselves.

Clients told them that hearing and seeing Walker talk about his diabetes so matter-of-factly helped motivate them to accept the situation that they were in and to do something about it.

"If there's any positive aspect to this whole thing, that's it," says Walker.

"Really Stupid"

Oh, sure, he's the model of acceptance now, but Walker didn't start out that way. Tested for diabetes in the spring of '91, he was declared glucose intolerant, and his doctor told him to keep an eye on it. He started losing weight, and about 6 months later the other tell-tale symptoms, like increased thirst, appeared. Walker figured he was developing diabetes, but still he didn't go to see his doctor.

"This is going to really sound stupid," says Walker. "I had for months been planning a short vacation with my dearest friends. We were celebrating some things, and I absolutely wanted to be able to enjoy it.

"I knew I was about to have my life changed to some degree, and I wanted to put it off until I got the trip out of the way. It was not smart, but at the time it was important to me. So I went and had a good time, and the first day back went into the hospital."

Well, yes, he did go to the hospital his first day back, but even then he pushed it pretty far.

"We were shooting our TV show with one of the local fire departments, showing how they rescue people. And I was so thirsty, so incredibly, unbelievably thirsty, and there wasn't any water. Here it is the fire department, and I'm saying, 'What do you mean you don't have any water?' and they said they didn't have any drinking water, and I said, 'What's the water quality of that hydrant over there?' They went over with the big hydrant wrench and opened it, and I just stood there with a cup and drank water out of the hydrant.

"I was in bad shape, but I got the show completed and then I just told everybody, 'I gotta go,' hopped in my car and drove straight to the hospital. When I got there, my blood sugar was 600 plus, and I gave myself my first injection an hour later."

He has had to change his lifestyle some, but he says he was never big on junk food, so diet isn't a big problem. And diabetes hasn't affected his favorite activity.

"I'm a golf fanatic, and since it's good exercise for burning off blood sugar, I've got a great excuse. If I'm not working or with my family, that's what I'd like most to be doing. Hitting the ball is incidental, I just enjoy the environment."

Although by his own admission he is just an adequate player, he has played on some of the top courses in the country. "When I stood on the 18th tee at Pebble Beach, I didn't even want to swing the club. I just wanted to stand there and look at it."

The Guy Who Didn't Start

Walker seems to have always been the regular guy who gets to do all the fun stuff. In school, in the small town of Dallas, Oregon, he got "OK" grades. On sports teams, he was "the guy who was good enough to make the team but didn't ever start. If they were one uniform short of having everyone look alike, I was the guy who looked different, the one who got last year's jersey." But after school, he would go to the local 1,000-watt radio station, which his father owned, and go on the air.

"I first went on the air when I was 13. My dad got the greatest kick out of telling people how he had to absolutely force me to open the microphone and give my name and the time.

"By the time I was in high school, I was on every afternoon after school."

Somehow, this regular guy got the girl, too. Barbara Steele, Honor Society and Homecoming Court member at Dallas High School, had recently broken up with her boyfriend and wasn't going to the Junior Prom. Her friends convinced Craig Walker, 130-pound geek (his description), to do the neighborly thing. He took Barbara to the dance; they recently celebrated their silver wedding anniversary, and have two children, Karen, 21, and Craig, 18.

Walker stumbled into a TV career in much the same way—by being the "well, he's available" guy in the right place at the right time. In 1972, he was working at a radio station that also owned a TV station. He had been at the station for 4 months when he was called to go in front of the cameras for the first time.

"The TV news director walked into the control room of the radio station and said, 'How'd you like to be on TV? I need a back-up sports guy.' I said, 'I don't have the slightest inkling about how to put a segment together,' and he said, 'Just be here Saturday and I'll show you how it's done.' Well, Saturday arrived and he didn't. So I ended up putting together something with the help of the other people in the newsroom."

Walker went on to anchor the sports regularly, and has been working on TV off and on ever since. He also hosted an audience participation show, and the now defunct *PM Magazine*. He's been co-host of *Good Evening* for 3 years.

Despite his success in TV, Walker says he'd never choose it over radio. "I do enjoy TV, but radio would win hands down. I'm a radio person. I love radio. It's so much more fun and fulfilling. The creative freedom of radio is everything to me. I don't consider my radio show a forum just for me to spout off. The number one priority is the listeners: what will interest, inform, or entertain them. But I can say, 'I'm going to talk about this because I think it's important,' and I don't have to worry about producers, directors, networks, commercial cues, or time constraints. I can't do that on TV."

Besides, he can't leave his radio family. "For a lot of people, probably most, I'm just a button on the radio," says Walker. "But there are others out there much more deeply involved."

Walker has a liver disease, and is waiting for a transplant. "That has caused an incredible outpouring of concern. I've gotten letters from many listeners that were unbelievably touching. I learned that I'm truly one of the closest people to them. I'm closer than family in some cases. It took me a while to grasp that, because I sit in a room and talk to myself."

Listeners sometimes call the station to complain when Walker goes on vacation, but when his pager goes off, telling him there's a liver for him, they'll forgive him his absence. As long as he comes back soon, to ease them into their day.

It's 7:20, 65 or 70 for highs today, it's gonna be a neat day....

Marie McCarren is associate editor of Diabetes Forecast.

Ken Finkelstein: Blue Ocean, Black Oil

by Marcia Levine Mazur

This article appeared in *Diabetes Forecast,* September 1992.

A midnight summons to help fight the world's largest oil spill helped Ken Finkelstein discover his lifelong career. Ken Finkelstein was a 21-year-old graduate student in geology when a midnight phone call changed his life. His professor, Miles Hayes, PhD, was on the line, and he had fast-breaking news. An oil tanker, the *Amoco Cadiz,* had just cracked apart in rough seas off the coast of France; thousands of barrels of crude oil were blackening the historic beaches of Brittany. Hayes had an offer. Would Finkelstein join him and the the rest of the American team who were flying over to help fight the flowing oil?

"Imagine being 21 and being invited to go to France the next day!" Finkelstein says.

He accepted but couldn't get back to sleep. Ken Finkelstein had a special concern. Although Hayes didn't know it at the time, 6 months earlier Finkelstein had been diagnosed with type 1 diabetes. He was still coming to terms with the startling news.

Before that, the Queens, N.Y., native, transplanted to the University of South Carolina graduate school, had been living life to the hilt. In fact, he remembers himself in those days as an "urban cowboy."

Then came urinary problems, fatigue, and the shocking diagnosis. Impossible, he thought. As far as he knew, no one in his family had diabetes, yet suddenly someone was telling him he'd be "sticking needles into himself" for the rest of his life.

"When you're 21, you think you're indestructible," he

recalls, "so when the doctor said I had diabetes, I told him, 'you've got the wrong guy!'"

Now the midnight call brought new concerns. Would his diabetes affect his work? Could he even get his syringes past French customs?

Syringes And Custom Officers

Finkelstein has learned a lot since that spring night in 1978. He knows now that if you take care of yourself, diabetes needn't stop you from working long days, catching last-minute flights, being dropped on remote beaches, or choosing an exciting profession.

He knows, too, that most customs officers, even in obscure backwaters of the globe, don't bat an eyelash over diabetes supplies.

Mopping up in the wake of the *Amoco Cadiz* taught Finkelstein something else, too. The oil-stained beaches of Brittany stirred him deeply and firmed his resolve to do what he could to control human insults to the Earth. In fact, that fouled coastline whetted his appetite for a new area of study—environmental science.

His friend Craig Shipp, now a research geologist with Shell Oil Company, puts it this way, "Ken picked up the environmental theme from day one and never let go."

"Actually," Finkelstein explains, "although the profession is called environmental science, it has no official name yet. It's a very new field, still mainly self-taught, and it brings together many scientific disciplines. That's one of the nice things about it."

Finkelstein returned to the States, finished his master's degree in coastal geology, took additional geology studies at the University of Maryland, then switched to geological oceanography for his doctorate from The College of William and Mary, Virginia Institute of Marine Sciences.

Overpowering

While investigating the world around him, Finkelstein also came to terms with the world inside himself, the world of diabetes. "You absolutely have no choice but to deal with it," he says. "I'm aware of it not only when I eat, but every time I even think of food, exercise, or travel. I find diabetes such an overpowering aspect of my life that learning to live with it has become relatively easy."

That approach was, literally, a lifesaver, once the midnight emergency phone calls became almost commonplace. Finkelstein was summoned to many oil spills, including the Haven spill in Italy, the World Prodigy spill off Narragansett Bay in Rhode Island, and the *Ixtoc* spill off the Yucatan Peninsula. That one reached all the way to Padre Island, Texas. His friend Shipp sums it up, "Wherever there was a major spill, Ken was there."

Even the ghost of the *Amoco Cadiz* sailed across his path again. In the late 70s, working part-time at the Research Planning Institute (RPI) in Columbia, South Carolina, he helped evaluate the lessons of that ill-fated vessel.

Swamped

Finkelstein's strangest call, though, was to a mangrove swamp in Puerto Rico. There, a wrecked barge called the *Peck Slip* had soaked the swamp with oil. Finkelstein and Shipp were sent to assess the damage.

"Working in the swamp was like being put down in a plate of spaghetti after someone poured steak sauce over it, then being asked to determine how much sauce was there," Shipp recalls.

Then came a providential assignment. Finkelstein, still working part time with RPI, conducted a U.S. National Oceanic and Atmospheric Administration (NOAA)-sponsored team to Alaska. Their goal: Map some of the coastal areas and estimate their vulnerability to oil spills.

Finkelstein explains. "Imagine a coastline with a lot of marshes. It's clear that spilled oil will stay longer there than on a rocky coastline with big waves splashing against it."

The location chosen for the study was uncanny. "As luck would have it," Finkelstein says, "we did our work in Prince William Sound, the spot where the *Exxon Valdez* did spill its oil some time later."

Largest Tanker Spill In U.S. History

Few people watching the late news March 24, 1989, can forget the name of the tanker that befouled Alaskan waters that night: the *Exxon Valdez*.

The tanker ripped into a reef 25 miles from Valdez, the southern terminal of the Alaskan oil pipeline. Before the spill was controlled, it gushed 11 million gallons of crude into an Eden of fish, birds, and other wildlife called Prince William Sound.

While the *Amoco Cadiz* off the coast of France remains the world's largest oil tanker spill, the *Exxon Valdez* is the largest oil tanker spill in U.S. history.

Such an enormous spill pulled scientists from a wide geographical area, and Finkelstein got the call in Boston. This time, though, he was not too surprised. By then he had signed on full time with NOAA, an agency that works closely with the U.S. Coast Guard to combat oil spills. Although he was investigating the catastrophic effects of marine pollution in New England, Finkelstein knew he'd be heading to Alaska as soon as he got word of the spill.

Onto The Beaches

With a complement of oceanographers, chemists, biologists, and geologists, Finkelstein was helicoptered onto the beaches of Prince William Sound. The group was to determine the location of the oil, calculate where it was headed, then advise where to rush protective measures.

The need was urgent. The *Exxon Valdez'* cargo had begun oozing into the clear, cold waters of the sound just 2 months before May 15, the date local sea lions and seals head for the beaches to bear their young. Wildlife experts knew which beaches the animals favored, but they didn't know which ones the oil was heading toward after it spilled.

"We didn't want those new babies to die because they were covered with oil," Finkelstein recalls.

The first few months in Alaska were chaotic for Finkelstein, but by the end of the summer, things were running smoothly.

Much of the newborn seal and sea lion population was saved. In fact, Finkelstein adds, "The only population of mammals really impacted were the sea otters. They use their fur as insulation, and when the oil got on the fur they died from the cold."

Low Tide

In 1978 and 1979, while Finkelstein was first coping with diabetes, he frequently was dropped onto Alaskan beaches alone or with only one or two others. He realized then that it was up to him to make sure he stayed in good health. Working in Alaska is no picnic for someone with type 1 diabetes.

The message was amplified by the *Exxon Valdez*. Although he came in with a larger group at that time, the scientists were determined to get the job done as quickly as possible. Since the Alaskan sun barely set at night, they worked nearly 18 hours at a stretch.

Finkelstein explains, "There are two low tides during the day, and we worked both of them, because at low tide we could see the whole beach."

That meant rolling out of their bunks about 4 a.m., working through the first low tide, waiting out high tide, getting back to business during the second low tide, then calling it a day—and night—about 10 p.m, only to repeat the schedule a few hours later, rested or not.

"I Am The Key"

"I realized how fully I was the key to my own good health," Finkelstein recalls. "Some of the others, for example, could go all day without food, but I had to be ready with my own peanut butter sandwiches and crackers."

Finkelstein carried his insulin, syringes, and blood-testing equipment wherever he went. "I overdid it with a double supply," he says, "but I knew that if something broke on that beach, I'd be out of luck."

He discovered, too, that it paid to be strong-willed. "When I was young I was shy about my diabetes. Now I just say, 'Wait a minute. I have to take a shot' or 'I have to eat something.' And people are always sympathetic. I'm not one to tell everybody I have diabetes, but when you're in the field, in a helicopter, on a research cruise, or doing two tides a day, you have to let the people you work with know in case you have a reaction."

Fortunately, Finkelstein has never had an insulin reaction while on an oil spill expedition. His only diabetes-related health problems have come when the disease delayed his recovery from other illnesses.

Although working in Alaska was especially difficult for Finkelstein, he found it extraordinarily rewarding. "It's just beautiful there," he says. "You see killer whales and soaring eagles, and when the salmon run upstream, they're so thick you can pick them out from a helicopter."

Moving On

By 1991, Finkelstein had been working for government agencies for more than 8 years, during which time he studied coastal trends and beach erosion for the Army Corps of Engineers Coastal Engineering Research Center at Ft. Belvoir, Virginia. (The Center is now located in Vicksburg, Mississippi.) He also worked at the Boston office of the NOAA. He had grown curious about life in the private sector, so, in 1991, Finkelstein joined Arthur D. Little, Inc., a consulting firm in Cambridge, Massachusetts, that works on environmental issues.

Married in 1987 to lawyer Lisa Alkon, Finkelstein now revels in married life and the joys of fatherhood. He dotes on the couple's 2-year-old daughter, Erica. "She's truly the apple of my eye," he says.

Finkelstein, who recently learned that a long-deceased grandparent also had diabetes, admits to keeping a close eye on Erica for signs of the disease; so far, fortunately, none have appeared.

Although Finkelstein no longer describes himself as a "cowboy," the joys of his life run deep. He has good control of his diabetes, works out with weights twice a week—"used to be three times," he confesses—plays on two summer softball teams, one for men and the other where Lisa is a teammate, and puts in some biking time. "But I wish I had more willpower with food," he adds.

A Message From Dr. Kenneth Finkelstein

People always ask me about the *Amoco Cadiz* or the *Exxon Valdez* oil spills. Of course, such spills grab the public's attention. But, except for inactive coastal environments, natural processes remove much of the oil from tanker spills, even those of catastrophic magnitudes. The oil breaks down, biodegrades, and eventually disappears. For instance, most of the visible signs of the Alaskan oil spill are gone now, and long-term effects to wildlife appear to be minimal.

In addition, oil from these spills covers only the surface of the water, while most fish are far underneath. Prince William Sound produced a record salmon catch the year after the *Exxon Valdez* spilled its cargo.

In many other of our waterways, there are fish with unacceptable amounts of contaminants in their tissues, although these contaminants were released 20 or more years ago and are now banned. In New York's Hudson River, striped bass continue to have levels of contaminants in their tissues that make them unfit for human consumption. And there is no end in sight. In New Bedford Harbor, Mass., the insult to the sediment deep under the water is so great it will be decades before it can again be utilized as a fishery habitat.

Clearly, the real harm to our marine environment is not the once-in-20-years oil spill, but the slow, insidious, continuous release of chemicals and sewage into our waters. Our waters suffer from decades (possibly a century or more) of abuse, particularly from persistent chemicals such as PCBs (used in transformers), pesticides, and heavy metals. Frequent, small doses of oil residue that wash off our city streets and enter nearby harbor waters also do much damage, along with antiquated sewage treatment facilities and indiscriminate harbor dumping.

Yet it's difficult to get the idea across that there is no quick fix. I think the U.S. Environmental Protection Agency's Superfund program to clean major toxic waste dumps is excellent. But cleaning waste that has accumulated over decades is a slow process—and a very expensive one. To fix Boston Harbor, for example, people's water bills must go up.

We must spend the time—and money—to clean up the devastation that has taken years to accumulate.

> And we must make sure no new chemicals, pollutants, or sewage, even as simple as a dumped beer can, enter our waters. We simply cannot treat these resources that way anymore. It is not the impressive oil tanker spills that have brought serious pollution to our waters. The cause is a lot closer to home.
>
> *For more information on solid waste disposal, including medical waste, contact the U.S. Environmental Protection Agency, RCRA, at (202) 260-9327, or the EPA Public Information Center at (202) 260-2080. Or, contact environmental organizations in your area.*

Then there are the pleasures of the part-time oceanography classes he teaches at Suffolk University in Boston, and the occasional talks he delivers on marine pollution to various organizations. Finkelstein also has published professional papers.

Perhaps his greatest happiness, though, comes at summertime, when he, Lisa, and Erica trek up to Edmund, Maine. There, he teaches senior citizens about the world's waters in a program run by the Elderhostel organization.

Whenever colleagues ask Finkelstein how he manages such a tight schedule while dealing with type 1 diabetes he tells them, "I don't think 'healthy' people realize how well they too would manage if serious illness should strike."

Finkelstein is glad that the world is facing up to some of its ecological problems in conferences such as the one recently held in Rio de Janiero. "But," he cautions, "the real work is usually done at smaller gatherings."

Now that he's a father, Finkelstein is pleased that his recent career move has allowed him to cut down on travel. "My wife works full time as an attorney, and it would be unfair for her to take care of Erica on her own while I am away," he says. "Still," he adds, "it's likely that when the world has another major oil spill, I'll be there!"

Marcia Levine Mazur is senior editor of Diabetes Forecast.

Bill Talbert: A Full Life of Service

by Joseph Wakelee-Lynch

This article appeared in *Diabetes Forecast,* August 1991.

Tell Bill Talbert he can't do something, and he'll try hard to do it, and do it better than anyone else.

Bill's experiences in life sharpened his strong sense of independence. He has competed in tennis matches, battled diabetes, or made business deals almost his entire life. During the 1940s and 1950s, Bill walked off United States tennis courts with 38 titles. At 72 years old, he was a successful businessman and a leader in the fight to cure and prevent diabetes. Bill's had type 1 diabetes for 63 years.

Howard Cosell, sports commentator for the American Broadcasting Company (ABC) and Bill's friend for almost 30 years, explained, "He had to be independent, because of all the obstacles he faced."

"I didn't want to be a slave to the diabetes," Bill remarked. "I needed the independence of dealing with it and not letting it run me."

"Retreat From Life"

Billy Talbert was born in Cincinnati, Ohio, on September 4, 1918. Like many other young boys, Billy dreamed of being a baseball player, just like his idols Ty Cobb and "Sunny" Jim Bottomley. But unlike most other young boys, he found out he had diabetes at the age of 10.

Because Billy's body couldn't convert sugar into energy, his doctor told his parents that Billy needed to avoid activities that demanded lots of energy. That meant no baseball and very little of any other sport. In other words, young Billy was grounded.

It was like "a forced retreat from life," Bill recalled in his autobiography, *Playing for Life* (Little, Brown and Company, 1958). So Billy took up marbles and soon became the best "shooter" in the neighborhood.

Billy's parents followed the best advice doctors could offer in the 1920s. Insulin had been discovered 7 years before, in 1921. There was still much to be learned about how insulin would affect the day-to-day lives of people with diabetes.

But one day, when Billy was 14 years old, his father came home from work with a gift that would change the boy's life. He pushed a tennis racket into young Bill's hands. His son needed something to do, the elder Talbert reasoned, because he was going stir crazy from inactivity. And their family doctor agreed.

On The Circuit

At first, Billy hardly knew what to do with a racket, but he practiced endlessly, and he learned. Young Talbert soon rose through the tennis ranks in Ohio. Then he joined a tennis circuit on the East Coast, accumulating wins and developing a reputation for smart, heady play.

"If there is such a thing as a natural—if tennis players are born, not made—then I wasn't it," Bill wrote in his book. "[I] didn't scare anybody just by walking onto the court. Nor did the ball explode when I hit it. I had all I could do to put a shot where I wanted it."

Bill Talbert built his career on his ability to place a tennis ball exactly where he wanted it. It was a skill that took him to the top of the tennis charts.

In 1946, he and Gardnar Mulloy were the first men's doubles team to win the U.S. Open three times. By 1950, Bill was rated the number 2 player at England's prestigious Wimbledon tournament. He and his partners also were rated number 1 in men's doubles and mixed doubles.

During his years on the tennis circuit, Bill was learning as much about managing his diabetes as about championship tennis. Planning his meals, of course, became crucial.

Through trial-and-error and advice from his doctor, Bill planned a "tennis diet." Breakfast was the time to eat slow-burning proteins in the form of lean ham, eggs, and milk. At noon, he ate more protein in the form of lean meat or fish, plus vegetables. Bill would also have some bread, potatoes, and sometimes a bit of ice cream to build up a carbohydrate reserve for an afternoon of tennis.

Then the low point of the day: late afternoon after a match. That was the time for some orange juice. But the "most important innovation of all," to Bill, was the late-night snack. Earlier, this would have been considered risky for a person with diabetes. But Bill consulted with his doctor and together they came up with a plan: He would consume a small portion of carbohydrate and slow-burning proteins in order to reduce the danger of an insulin reaction by giving the insulin something to work on overnight. "A sandwich or crackers and a glass of milk became a bedtime ritual with me," he recalled.

Game And Health Strategies

But Bill admits he struggled to maintain control of his diabetes. "I hadn't really mastered diabetes," Bill wrote in his autobiography, "I had only survived it, day by day."

"There were times," he said, "when I stretched it too much and thought that nothing could happen to me and I could do whatever I pleased. And I got myself into some trouble."

One incident took place in 1949. Bill faced Pancho Gonzales, the U.S. champion at the time, with the winner to take the Southampton Trophy. Bill started strong, winning the first set and taking the lead. But Gonzales came back, winning the next two. Bill was not only playing badly, he seemed more out of control with each point.

With Gonzales threatening to win the fourth set and the match, Bill's friend Mulloy, watching from the stands, realized the problem: Bill was having an insulin reaction. Mulloy rushed to courtside with a glass of water mixed with sugar. Bill downed it, recovered quickly, and almost without error won the remaining points and took home the trophy.

With experience, Bill began combining his diabetes plan with his game plan. He devised strategies that made the most of his physical abilities and exploited his opponents' weaknesses.

Just before the start of a tournament, for example, Bill would study the schedule of matches to see if his opponents were power players or control players.

He couldn't afford to let the players with big, powerful serves set the pace of the match—Talbert wasn't strong enough to play their power game. Instead, he had to confuse them, change the speed of his shots, and force a slower tempo than they liked. For that, Bill had to pace himself, conserving his energy.

But, sometimes, Bill faced opponents whose strengths mirrored his own: accuracy and control of the tempo. Again, he'd store up energy, and he'd practice less so he wouldn't be tired when the match started. Bill tried to make sure the control players didn't keep him on the court too long. He'd try to win these games as fast as he could.

In the end, Bill was adjusting his diet, his practice schedule, and his game strategy all at the same time. "At each tournament," Bill remembered, "when I walked onto the court for my opening round of play, I wasn't just starting a match, I was pursuing a health campaign."

After The Big Time

Although Bill's ability to manage diabetes seemed to improve along with his game, a trip to Australia opened his eyes to important work he would do helping others once he left "the big time" of championship tennis.

Talbert was in Melbourne with the U.S. Davis Cup team. When a journalist reported Bill's disease, letters and phone calls streamed in, asking Bill to give tennis exhibitions to Australian children with diabetes. Although he'd rarely been involved with this kind of work at home, he went anyway.

After returning to the United States, Bill realized that even though he was a hero to the children at the Australian clinics, he actually had been trying his hardest to "run" from his disease. Each victory was a way of becoming independent from diabetes, as if he could cure his diabetes with greater doses of trophies.

The second thing Bill realized was that he enjoyed working with kids immensely. He joked, teased, and cajoled, always urging the children to keep their diabetes in control and not to stop pursuing their dreams. "It made me realize I had an opportunity to help people," Bill recalled more than 40 years later, "and that I liked helping people."

Winning With Service

Helping people, in fact, has almost been Bill's full-time occupation since leaving the championship tennis circuit. And he continues to enjoy a special relationship with children.

For the last 45 years, Bill has worked with the ADA New York Downstate Affiliate at its annual diabetes camp, known as Camp NYDA. The camp's tennis court is named after him. Lynne Perry, executive director of the affiliate, said, "You'd think that a man of Talbert's age would be out of touch with kids today. But the kids are enthralled by him…kids who love the Teenage Mutant Ninja Turtles really respond to this man."

Bill also speaks frequently to groups and corresponds with young people, including tennis players. In 1990, his contributions were recognized by the ADA when he was awarded the Wendell Mayes, Jr., Medal "for outstanding volunteer service in the cause of diabetes."

Bill kept his hand in tennis long after he stopped playing at the top level. From 1953 to 1957 he captained the U.S. Davis Cup team, and for 15 years he was the director of the U.S. Open Tennis Championships in Forest Hills, New York. Talbert has also written seven books, most of them manuals on playing the game.

In 1960, Bill experienced one of those rare coincidences when a boyhood dream and adult work come together. Bill was asked to talk to a legendary ex-baseball player who'd been diagnosed with diabetes. It was Bill's childhood idol, Ty Cobb. Bill left Cobb with a copy of his book, which the ex-ballplayer found "enlightening," and he sent Bill a warm, appreciative letter in response.

Today, Bill still maintains a demanding pace of life. With his wife, Nancy, to whom he's been married for 43 years, Bill lives in New York City. Bill walks 3 to 4 miles a day; he plays golf 18 holes at a time. He weighs 160 pounds, just as he did at the top of his game. And he stopped playing tennis only 4 years ago.

Bill is now an executive vice-president of the American Bank Note Company, which engraves and prints stock certificates, bonds, traveler's checks, stamps, or other valuable documents. As he is in his personal life, so he is professionally: "Independence is a very, very important thing to me, and it has determined the way I've worked for 43 years."

Bill takes insulin once a day—in the morning. (Editor's Note: The majority of people with diabetes need more than one insulin injection per day.) He eats three meals a day: a light breakfast of orange juice and a piece of toast; a lunch of chicken vegetable soup and salad; and for dinner, a piece of fish or chicken or sometimes a steak or pasta.

Now, 63 years after being diagnosed with diabetes, Bill has proved that no one with diabetes has to begin a "full retreat from life." In fact, his example, coming so soon after insulin's discovery, has demonstrated that many people with the disease can live as actively as others.

As for Bill himself, he reflects on decades of athletics, business, and service. His greatest accomplishment?

"My career in tennis certainly provided a lot of success for me," Bill suggested.

But he added, "My greatest accomplishment, I guess, is that I have survived as long as I have."

Joe Wakelee-Lynch is a freelance writer who was formerly associate editor of Diabetes Forecast.

Bret Michaels: Making Music

by Marcia Levine Mazur

This article appeared in *Diabetes Forecast,* September 1989.

Rock star Bret Michaels is in love...with life, music, and health. He pours his passion into his songs, and millions of fans respond to his call.

Bret was the main ingredient, the frontman, of the rock group Poison. The Poison four—singer Bret Michaels, guitarist C.C. DeVille, drummer Rikki Rockett, and bassist Bobby Dall—criss-crossed the country in the late 1980s exploding their heavy metal sound before screaming audiences in sold-out concerts from Boston to Los Angeles. Then they carried their powerful potion to Australia and Japan.

But March 1986 was their magic month. That's when Poison brought out *Look What the Cat Dragged In,* their first album and their rocket to that sweet stratosphere where records go platinum. *Cat* sold 3 million in the United States alone, with a big play on the single "Talk Dirty to Me." Second album sales of *Open Up and Say...Ahh!,* out in April 1988, burst the 5 million mark here, again shooting singles centerstage, "Your Momma Don't Dance," "Fallen Angel," "Nothin' But A Good Time," and Bret's own, "Every Rose Has Its Thorn."

Bret knows about those thorns. The songwriter/singer, who turned 26 on March 15, 1989, has had type 1 diabetes since he was 6.

Although he and the band spent hours perfecting their music, Bret is almost as intense about diabetes. "I test anywhere from 6 to 10 times a day," he says. "Before the show and afterwards. I have to know where my sugars are at all times, because I have such a weird schedule."

His home on a rolling tour bus didn't contribute to clock-careful control. Wheeling into towns at dawn or midnight, frenetic performances, backstage parties kept Bret from always maintaining a routine diabetes regimen. But he recommends it to others.

"The more scheduled you can be, the better you control your diabetes, the better off you are," he says. "Unfortunately, I lead an irregular life. There's no schedule. But I do the best I can. I base my diabetes care according to when I eat, but some days I get up at 9, some days at 1. But whenever I wake up I eat a good breakfast. And I have a good dinner. Then I don't eat too much after that because it slows me down onstage."

Although Bret's great grandmother, grandmother, and several aunts and uncles had diabetes, the disease was new to the first-grader. "I couldn't understand why I had it. As I grew up, I'd look at other kids doing what I was doing, maybe playing football, only I was feeling funny and they weren't," he remembers.

"Of course it was a shock to my family. Of course we cried about it. After all, here's this 6-year-old kid who has to take shots every day."

Bret handled the injections well, but learned that non-physical problems come from other people's view of the disease. He credits his mom, Marjorie, and dad, Wally, for that approach. "They're divorced now, but they have each been very supportive of me," Bret says.

"I was never taught to be embarrassed or feel different. The way I act, you would never know I have diabetes unless I have a reaction."

Diabetes didn't stop the young Bret any more than it slows the rock star. His secret is attitude. "I accept the fact that I have diabetes. Otherwise, I try to make my life as normal as possible. It's like accepting anything. You have to know the rules. Sure, sometimes you break rules. But you have to know them before you can break them."

A Reason To Wake Up

Diabetes wasn't the only factor in young Bret's life. There was music. "To some people music is just to listen to. To me, it was something that made me feel great."

Music has done more than that. It has given Bret purpose. "I am one of those people who believes you need a reason to wake up in the morning, whether to work or play," he explains.

Music has always been his "something." "I express the way I feel though music. To me, it's a kind of poetry. It's a great feeling."

That great feeling landed Bret in his first band before he hit the seventh grade. "They were garage bands. You got together in someone's garage and you figured the songs out from records."

Although he took vocal, guitar, and harmonica lessons as a youngster, Bret picked up most of his musical skills on his own. And he daydreamed of fame.

"One of my first songs, 'Cry Tough' was about believing in yourself. You have to believe in yourself in order to achieve anything."

Bret believed. "When I was in front of my mirror, all alone in my room with my stereo loud, I dreamed of being famous. If I wasn't here, I'd still be in my room dreaming. Dreaming is good."

While he dreamed at home in Pennsylvania, he listened to groups like AC/DC, Kiss, the Beatles, Rolling Stones, Led Zeppelin, even folk music.

And he acted like a lot of other teenagers. "I gave my folks a hard time when I was growing up," he recalls. "I don't think my parents appreciated my hair. It was always long. And I ran away from home. You know, 'Hey, you won't give me the car tonight. Okay, I'm running away from home.'" He also recalls that running away from problems never solved them.

"But I have a great family," Bret adds. "Great relatives. Good friends. It's nice to know that." Bret has two sisters, Michelle, production assistant for Poison and sometime worker with the group Whitesnake, and 15-year-old Nicole, still in school.

On To L.A.

In the early 1980s Bret and his musician friends packed up their young band and struck out for California.

Why "Poison"?

Bret explains: "When we played in Pennsylvania they said we were poisoning the youth of America. We decided, 'If we're poison, so be it.'"

But in Los Angeles, the dream twisted into a nightmare. Bret recalls, "We lived in a busted warehouse. It was really horrible. Before we left Pennsylvania I had a job. I was on my own. I wasn't used to warehouse living." Neither was his diabetes.

"The band kept an eye on me, and they got me out of trouble a number of times when I was having an insulin reaction. Only once did I pass out onstage. Toward the beginning of my career, I thought I didn't need to take precautions. I got so low I started feeling funny, and while I was trying to get to the side of the stage, I just went unconscious," Bret recalls. "I'm much more careful about myself now," he adds.

The group was barely surviving in Los Angeles. Still, they acquired guitarist C.C. DeVille there. "He and I had an argument when we first met," Bret recalls. "He said his band was better. I said mine was. Pretty soon he was in mine."

Poison scrambled to be noticed. They toured with groups like Ratt, Cinderella, and singer David Lee Roth. Poison members distributed their own flyers, wrote music, attracted attention, and pushed at the magic door to success.

Finding Fame

After 3 years of trying, the door opened. Their dues paid, Poison was a headliner. Finally, they could blast out their music, Bret romping onstage, long streaming locks flaring around his shoulders as he punched out their songs to the crowds who came now just for them.

The four Poison pals established an identity with an outrageous style of striking female makeup, motorcycles, skateboards, racing bikes, legendary parties, and tattoos.

But Bret is clear about the reason for their musical success. "We took off because our band is based on heart," he explains. "If you don't have the feelings, you are not going to project them. Some bands work just to have an album or video. But if you're in the business just to get famous, you won't sound the same. I have the fame. But I still want to play my kind of music."

His kind of music? "Call us heavy metal, hard rock, rock and roll, pop rock, glam rock, whatever you like. Every band has a fingerprint. I am different, say, from Bon Jovi because I have different ideas, different influences. In music, all those differences spill out."

Bret glories in the sacks of mail, the packs of screaming fans. The feeling is mutual. Katherine and Rebecca Nykwest of Alexandria, Virginia, speak for the legions of teens who paper their walls with Poison pictures. "We've been fans ever since 'Talk Dirty To Me,'" Katy and Becky remember. The sisters love Poison because "they're cute, their music is fun, and some of their songs have pretty deep meaning."

But Bret's tightest bond may be with the fans who have diabetes and other physical challenges. Fifteen-year-old Kiva Kamerling of Chestnut Hill, Massachusetts, who has had diabetes since she was 4, is still glowing from the night Bret singled her out from a backstage crowd. She displays their photo together to prove it. Kiva thinks Bret knew from other sources that she had diabetes. "He's an inspiration to me," Kiva says.

Still, Poison isn't everyone's cup of tea. The manic volume and insistent beat of metallic rock don't go down well with parents or neighbors who find that no wall or door will shut it out.

Others feel some of Poison's pranks need a warning label. Philip Levy, MD, editor in chief of *Diabetes Forecast* in 1989, cautioned that, although tattoos aren't necessarily harmful for people with diabetes, skin infections can occur more frequently when you have diabetes, making tattoos somewhat risky. Also, tattoos are permanent; attempts at removal can be unsuccessful and painful, sometimes even requiring skin grafting with extensive scarring.

Bret agrees his lusty lifestyle isn't for everyone. "People should act their own way. Some kids are fast. Some are slow. I may have tattoos, but I'm not telling anyone else to get them."

"I Like Feeling Healthy"

Though he's a shocker to some adults, he offers a message to post-teens who learn they have diabetes. "It's rough. You live most of your life, then suddenly, you've got this disease. So sit down, cry, punch a bag, slam a door, bust a window, knock a hole in the wall—whatever it takes that day to get over it. Then realize you have diabetes and get on taking care of yourself."

To young people he advocates a life without fear. "Some of the kids I meet with diabetes are so scared. I want to tell them it's OK to be scared, but you can't live in fear. You can't just say, 'Oh, God, I have diabetes. I can't do anything.' I wish they'd train kids not to be afraid, but to be prepared.

"Listen, you got to go out and get a grip on life and do the best you can. Just take care of yourself, and always be prepared wherever you go, whatever you're doing, partying or what. Make sure your friends know you have diabetes. Tell them the symptoms to look for, and exactly what to do if you don't look or act right. Remember, you are worthwhile to yourself and to your friends. If you can't tell them you have diabetes, if they won't help you out, then they're not your friends.

"I keep glucose with me at all times. Wherever I am, I make sure someone knows what to do if I have a low blood sugar reaction.

"Then I think kids with diabetes should go on and do the usual things all kids do, skateboarding, motorcycling, basketball, whatever."

At a shade under 5 feet 10 inches and 135 pounds, Bret proves his own attraction to action. "I do most any kind of exercise. I do martial arts every day. I like to do things that are demanding because they keep me in good shape." He adds, "I like feeling as healthy as I can. I watch my diet, I exercise, and I don't feel it's a sin to party. I'm just always prepared."

But music is still Bret's reason for getting up in the morning. "I love what I do. Although it's not an easy life—I've been on the road since April 1988—there's no greater high than being onstage hearing the screams. I'm also learning to play piano and sax now, and I love being on the move, seeing different cities. The places I've traveled!

"I know one day the fame will go. There are a lot of good bands out there. But I will keep on playing my music. I played my music before anyone knew who I was; I'll play it long after anyone cares. I can't complain. You do your thing as long as you feel good doing it. Then you get a little older, and maybe you want to settle. Life goes through phases," he says.

"I am emotional. I live with my heart. I see a mother on TV who loses her son to a drunk driver, and I get mad. But emotion makes me turn around and fight that much harder. I can be moody, too. I know the diabetes brings mood changes and that's another reason I try to keep it under control."

Bret has one final word. "I don't want people to think I am just this happy-go-lucky, or that nothing bad ever happened to me. A lot goes wrong in my life, and I can get quite stressed. That's why I wrote a song like 'Rose.' And after all, taking two shots a day isn't easy. But I try to turn things around, to make everything as positive as I can. It's good to know you are making the best of your life.

"And," he adds, "I'm always looking for love."

Marcia Levine Mazur is senior editor of Diabetes Forecast.

Serena Shapiro: A Special Kind of Service

by Marie McCarren

This article appeared in *Diabetes Forecast,* October 1992.

Serena Shapiro doesn't have many long conversations at parties. "When I say I'm a hospice social worker, there's no further conversation," says Shapiro, of Brookline, Massachusetts. "Or they'll say to me, 'That must be the most depressing job in the whole world.'"

Hospice professionals provide medical and emotional support to people who are dying. Shapiro, 36, has been working with people who are terminally ill for 3 years now, and she doesn't find it a bit depressing. In fact, she says her work acts as an antidote to the violence she reads about every day.

"You pick up the daily paper and the front page is: This person was murdered, this one was robbed. I see the flip side of humanity. I see a tremendous spirit and caring and compassion among human beings in my work. I do see a lot of sadness, but I also see incredible courage and fortitude."

From Patient To Counselor

Shapiro's own experiences in hospitals led her to a career in hospice. She was diagnosed with type 1 diabetes when she was a freshman at Brandeis University in Waltham, Massachusetts. She found out that the health care system, with its chronic understaffing and dependence on insurance, can sometimes be dehumanizing for both staff and patients.

"There were situations where I was just not treated as if I were a person. I was Insulin + Food + Exercise = Blood sugar: a number. I found something missing. Sensitivity sometimes gets lost."

As a social worker at Hospice of Cambridge, in Cambridge, Massachusetts, Shapiro makes sure her clients never feel like just a number. She works as part of a team of doctors, nurses, and home health aides upholding the ideals of hospice: "Our philosophy is that people should have as much control over their situation as possible, that they be as physically comfortable as possible, and that they be emotionally and spiritually at peace."

Shapiro does supportive counseling with people who, according to doctors' estimates, have less than 6 months to live. "I give patients emotional support and help them maintain their sense of spiritual dignity.

"I do life review with people. It's important to be able to reflect back on your life and hold onto what was good," she says. "Many people will reflect on their life and pull out very poignant, wonderful memories and fine achievements. Sometimes people look back with much regret, at things they wish they had done differently, and that's OK, too."

Dignity In Death

Even before Shapiro decided on a career in hospice, she was helping people come to terms with death. When she was diagnosed with diabetes, she was working toward her bachelor's degree in Judaic Studies. She spent her junior year studying in Israel. While there, she volunteered in the research department of a museum and memorial for the 6 million Jews who were killed in death camps during the Holocaust of World War II.

"I wanted to give honor to those who were killed," she says. "They don't even have graves." Shapiro has a personal interest: Her father, Leonard, was a Holocaust survivor. He spent a year in hiding when he was a young teen, in what is now Poland, and escaped to the United States with his parents and sister.

Shapiro says her father didn't talk about his experiences living under Nazi rule, but just knowing that he was there during those terrible times had a profound influence on her life. After she earned her bachelor's degree from Brandeis, she was set to return to Israel for graduate school. She planned to do research on the Holocaust, to keep the memory alive. "As this generation dies off, people will forget what happened," says Shapiro. "I believe in the old adage that if you forget history, you are destined to repeat it."

But just before she left for Israel, her father died suddenly. She didn't want to leave the country so soon after his death and so she took a job at the Joslin Diabetes Center, on a research project. She felt the work was important, but the lab setting didn't satisfy her need for the human element.

"It wasn't enough for me to know that my work would eventually benefit someone with diabetes," says Shapiro. "I wanted to work directly with people who were sick." She got a master's degree in social work from Boston University and found her niche working with people who were terminally ill.

Above And Beyond

Most of her clients have cancer; about a quarter have AIDS. Last year the AIDS Action Committee of Massachusetts honored Shapiro for her "extraordinary work in the AIDS effort." One reason she was honored involved her above-and-beyond battle to get a Haitian boy a visa to visit his mother in the States. The 12-year-old boy got his visa, and was able to see his mother before she died of AIDS.

Concern with the patient's family is one of the ways social work differs from other health care professions. "It's a holistic view," says Shapiro. "We look at the entire family environment, and that can include not only blood relatives, but also friends and neighbors." Shapiro counsels her clients as they approach death, as well as their families. Following a death, she offers bereavement support to surviving family members for 1 year, or longer, if necessary.

"In the aftermath, the families need reassurance that they did all they could. They often say, 'If I had only done this or that, John would be alive.' They are some-times angry at their relative who died for not going to the doctor sooner. They need support while they are grieving." Shapiro helps them move forward in the heal-ing process.

Debbie Manning, of Somerville, Massachusetts, says tak-ing care of her dying father would have been a lot harder without Shapiro. "She was like our guardian angel," says Manning. "We would have walked the road anyway—we had to—but she made it a lot easier. She'd praise us, make us feel we could keep going—'You have done wonders. I know how hard it is.' We knew we were doing a hard job, but it's nice to hear someone say it.

"Sometimes she'd call and all I did was cry—no words came out. She'd tell me, 'It's OK to feel this way.' She pulled us all together. She has a calm about her, an inner peace. She makes you feel the way she is—tranquil.

"She'd call us even when she was off duty. After my father died, she didn't forget us. She's still there for us. She really cares."

Dealing With Diabetes

Shapiro says that having diabetes has helped her in her work. "I will never know what they are going through, but I can empathize because I know what it feels like to have a chronic illness."

Shapiro has some complications due to her diabetes, most recently neuropathic pain. "It's really frightening to me. That's what really gets my spirit down, and I have to work to keep it up.

"But at this point in my life, the day-to-day care of my diabetes is not a thorn in my side. There have been times when I struggled with it. It has given me an immense amount of challenge. It has also given me a way of looking at life, a sense of mortality, knowing that I literally have control over my life."

She has used an insulin pump for 5 years, in what she calls a love-hate relationship. "The pump takes a lot more work, and it's expensive to run, but it gives me far better control than I ever had with multiple injections. But to be attached to a box every minute, 24 hours a day, can really get obnoxious after a while.

"Little things frustrate me: If I want to wear a dress, I have to figure out where I want to wear the pump. I go to the beach—am I going to go into the water and take it off and leave it in my bag on the beach? Or am I not going to go in the water?"

Hospice: What It Is, *Where* To Go

The term *hospice* stems from medieval times, when it was used to describe a place of shelter for sick travelers. Hospice was first used to describe specialized care for dying patients in 1967, when Dr. Cicily Saunders established St. Christopher's Hospice in England.

Today, hospice care is provided to people who can no longer benefit from treatment aimed at a cure. Hospice treats the person, not the disease. The goal is to neither hasten nor postpone death, but to manage pain and symptoms so the patient's last days are spent with dignity.

Care is provided by a hospice team—physicians, nurses, counselors, therapists, aides, and volunteers—in homes, hospitals, or freestanding hospice clinics. Help and support are available to the patient and family 24 hours a day.

Hospice care is covered under most private insurance plans. It is also covered by Medicaid in some states, and by Medicare (call your U.S. Department of Health and Human Services and ask for publication HCFA 02154 "Medicare: Hospice Benefits").

There are about 1,800 hospice programs in the United States. If you wish to find out if there is a hospice in your area, ask your doctor, or a member of the clergy, or call the nearest hospital, home health agency, or visiting nurses' association. About 25 states now have licensing requirements for hospices; check with the health department in your state. Medicare has certification requirements.

This information was provided by the nonprofit National Hospice Organization. You can contact them for information and referrals at 1901 N. Moore St., Suite 901, Arlington, VA 22209, or call their Hospice Help Line: (800) 658-8898.

Despite her complications, she doesn't feel that the pump has let her down. "It's not a given that you won't get complications if you take care of yourself. There may be inherent weaknesses. Still, I feel better on the pump, and it gives me much more freedom on a day-to-day basis."

Regular exercise is an important part of her life, and she spends most of her vacations hiking and camping. She also sticks to a balanced, no-meat diet. While she eats this way for health reasons—the diet helps her battle high cholesterol—she first adopted this diet simply because it was easier. When she was living in Israel, she was keeping kosher. Part of keeping kosher means having separate dishes and cooking utensils for meat and dairy products. "It became simpler not to have meat dishes," says Shapiro. Shapiro's deep faith sustains her during hard times. "I believe in God. I believe in the power of prayer, not because I believe that if I pray to God, God will change my situation. When I pray, I feel that I am not alone, that I have more strength."

Her clients also help her. "I see people going through very difficult situations, so I feel that I can contend with whatever I need to. The things I draw on are: prayer—the serenity prayer is sort of the foundation of my life, the memory of my father, and the courage of my patients."

Shapiro says she draws on the things that bring her pleasure: hiking, gardening, and playing the piano. She was taught piano by a professional: her mother, whom Shapiro describes as a "vivacious, incredible woman."

"I don't let my diabetes stand as the one thing that's always there. There's a lot more to life than an insulin pump and needles and pills," Shapiro says. "Those are ways to get to life, but it's not the central focus of my life."

Marie McCarren is associate editor of Diabetes Forecast.

Joseph Jones: Taking Charge

by Marie McCarren

This article appeared in *Diabetes Forecast,* May 1993.

Joseph Jones is hooked on his city: "I've traveled all over the United States, and I haven't found any city better than this." He's talking about Detroit.

Save your breath—he knows people need a little convincing about the virtues of Detroit, and he's ready: "It's a good city. They have good housing here, at a reasonable price, and most of the people are quite decent.

"If you're looking for the bad things about Detroit, the news media will help you. That's all they cover—the crime element. Sure, there are places in the city that I don't go, but normally, I have no problem in the city."

Jones knows his city isn't perfect, and he's working on it. He helped organize the Detroit Recreational Swim Club, which offers children and youths, from just-toilet-trained to age 18, a chance to compete in statewide meets. In 1988, the city council honored Jones with The Spirit of Detroit award "in recognition of exceptional achievement, outstanding leadership, and dedication to improve the quality of life" for his work with the swim club.

Jones also keeps a fatherly eye on the goings-on of his city and doesn't hesitate to voice his opinion at city council meetings if he thinks the politicians are headed in the wrong direction. He believes the small, everyday efforts of average citizens will add up to make a big difference, and will keep his hometown the best city in the U.S.

Poor And Tough

"We didn't live in the best neighborhood," Jones, 64, says of his childhood home. "In fact, I think we lived in the roughest neighborhood in the Detroit area. But you could leave your door open. Now you lock your door no matter what neighborhood you live in.

"If you had a problem you could usually handle it with fists. The worst thing that could happen to you when I was growing up was you might get cut. They didn't have gun control, but they had a form of gun control—nobody had them. Now everybody's got a gun, and they use them. People are more callous.

"It was poor and it was a tough neighborhood, but out of that neighborhood, a lot of good people came. There was more guidance then, more parents involved."

Jones' father died when Jones was 13; his mother, he says, kept him from getting involved with the criminal element.

"My mother was a strong woman. There were certain rules that you had to live by. We lived in a four-flat. My mother made us get up every morning and scrub the house, and it would be shining. She said, 'There's nothing in the house, but people will be dropping by and we don't want to create a bad impression.' That was a value of my mother's: Even if we don't have anything, it's going to be clean.

"The neighbors were different back then, too—they would inform on you. They would call before you got home: 'I saw Joseph doing such-and-such, at such-and-such a place.' When I got home, I caught hell. If I said the neighbor was lying, my mother would say, 'She wouldn't lie.'

"Now if you call a neighbor, they say, 'You don't need to tell me about my kid.' So you don't do it. If you inform on them, it's to the police directly."

Jones played football and ran track in high school. After he graduated from Northwest High, he put in 2 years as a Navy seaman, as World War II was nearing its end. "I saw real poverty when I was in the Navy," Jones says of his tours in the Caribbean. "It was the kings, the queens, and the paupers. Suddenly the way I lived wasn't looking so bad."

Jones couldn't afford college, and didn't need it to make a living. After he got out of the Navy, he worked as a machine operator for DeSoto and Cadillac for 6 years.

In the early '50s, he joined the United States Postal Service, working as a mail carrier and training other carriers. In 1977, when he was 48, he was promoted to management. But as his career went on an upswing, his health went down: In 1980, he was diagnosed with type 2 diabetes.

"As long as I was a carrier," says Jones, "I never had any problems, because I walked every day, at least 5 miles, up and down steps. After I went into management, my habits changed, and I began to have some problems."

Life Changes

At the time, Jones didn't know he had a family history of diabetes and was surprised at the diagnosis. "I had never had any illness before, and I thought they had made some kind of mistake."

But there was no mistake, so Jones made changes right away. When he was young, his mother kept him from the streets; now, diabetes keeps him from what he calls his street life, which means no more hanging out with the guys, drinking his way from club to club.

"I never met a stranger till I got diabetes," he says. "Anyone I met was a friend. If they wanted to drink, it was cool. If it was eating time, that was cool too.

"Diabetes curtailed my street life. I started picking my friends and my situations. If you hang out with people who are alcohol drinkers, they seem, when you're not drinking, to kind of get on your nerves. They get obnoxious, and you don't seem to have a great deal in common.

"So your life changes. But I have my family and long-standing friends, and I don't have any problem being lonely." Jones and his wife, Carrie, have three grown children, Joseph, Floyd, and Teri, and a teenage son, Jason, 15, who lives at home.

Jones is also raising his 11-year-old grandson, Joseph Jones IV, using the firm approach he learned from his mother. When young Joseph came to live with Jones 2 years ago, he had a tendency to misbehave. Strict discipline put Joseph on the straight and narrow at home, but school was another matter.

"He's a bright kid, but he was doing poorly in school, so I put him under what I call room arrest. He came home, did his homework, went to his room. No television, just a book if he wanted to read. It took 3 months before he finally realized he had to behave in school. On his last report card he got one C, all the rest As and Bs. It worked, because I made him accountable for his own actions.

"It's Up To Me"

Jones uses the same standards for himself. He—not his doctor, his friends, or Carrie—is accountable for keeping his diabetes under control.

"The doctor can only tell me what he advises—it's up to me to maintain."

Jones retired from the Postal Service in 1983 ("the other carriers said I really retired when I went into management") and has gone back to his pre-management roots—he walks, even during Detroit's sometimes bitterly cold winters.

"The weather can always be taken care of when you have your own transportation. I can always drive to a mall. It doesn't take a great deal of walking; I usually do 30 minutes. When I walk on a daily basis, I notice a difference in my wind and so forth.

"But I do get lazy. I find any excuse that works—it's cold, it's raining. Not that I'm looking for them, I just happen to find them. I have to be jolted. I become more and more lax, and then I realize—hey wait a minute, my condition is deteriorating, I have to start walking."

For A Good Cause...

He has taken control of his diet, in his own fashion. "My son doesn't have an eating problem, so my wife caters to his eating habits, not mine. That's her choice. It's my choice whether I eat it or not. I eat around what she cooks. She says if I don't like it, I can cook. Her nature is 'You're grown, you have to take care of yourself.'"

True to his nature, Jones is doing his bit to advance diabetes research. He has volunteered as a research subject several times. "I'm retired, so I'm available," he says.

For one of the trials, Jones was housed at a motel attached to the University of Michigan Medical Center and ate a very-low-calorie diet ("almost water, really") for a week. "I was a guest guinea pig," says Jones. But he was glad to do it. "I always learned something about my diabetic condition during these studies, and the researchers learned something from me."

Jones recently started using insulin, because he found his blood sugars stayed high even when he fasted. He's pleased he was able to go without insulin for 12 years after his diagnosis, though he feels he could have gone longer without insulin if he had controlled his diet better.

"I've never cooked, and there lies the problem. I imagine I could learn how to cook—I can read. But I don't have any patience for it. I just don't think a person should spend all day trying to fix food. There are too many other things to do. So I just eat around what's around."

Jones, with his typical easy-going attitude, has advice for people looking for ways to socialize with friends without it affecting their diabetes control: "If someone insists on you having a drink, let him pour it. Then, waste it. It's not your money—don't worry about it. If they insist that you eat, you can let them put the food on the plate and don't eat it. It's up to you whether you go the last step.

"We all live with choices. You have to make the choices that are best for you."

Marie McCarren is associate editor of Diabetes Forecast.

Rick Mystrom: Business Boom Alaska Style

by Roger Doughty

This article appeared in *Diabetes Forecast,* April 1997.

Add to the list of leading Alaskan exports—fur, fish, fuel, and frequent forays of ice-cold air—the name of Rick Mystrom, melodious-voiced mayor of Anchorage, and that city's ambassador extraordinaire to the world-at-large.

Mystrom, a 6-foot 3-inch super salesman and former advertising agency owner, will go anywhere to entice a company to bring its business to Alaska's most heavily populated city or to peddle his town's products. Point to just about any place on the map—be it Tupelo or Tokyo—and chances are Mystrom has been there, or will be soon, singing the praises of his favorite city.

Anchorage has a lot to offer, and Mystrom, armed with enormous enthusiasm and his ever-present insulin pump, spends much of his time offering it to Fortune 500 CEOs, heads of government, and other potential buyers around the globe. "I don't actually cut many deals," he says, "but where deals are in the works, I'm there to assure people that we're a business-oriented community and that the mayor's office will be there to make sure things work smoothly."

On the home front, Mystrom puts his skills to work inspiring his staff, conversing with constituents, volunteering his time and talents to worthy organizations, such as the ADA Alaska Affiliate, and stalking submarine-sized salmon. If there's a better job to be had, Mystrom can't imagine what it could be.

Anchorage

While many of Mystrom's daily duties are typical of those performed by other mayors, Anchorage has a chilly Camelot quality about it that makes even the most mundane matters seem magical. It's not just another city, say those who live there, it's an independent entity frozen to the edge of eternity. With 270,000 residents, the city is home to half the state's population. As Mystrom explains it, "There's Anchorage, then there's nothing for 1,500 miles. We're not near anything. Isolation is what defines our city."

Mystrom admits that isolation is "both a plus and a minus," but the majority of those who choose to live in this free-spirited community, where the sun rarely sets in summer and seldom shines in December, thrive on it. Having wilderness just outside their doors suits these fiercely independent urban woodsfolk just fine. For them, a little civilization goes a long way.

About 1,000 moose wander around town during winter, protected from hunters by city ordinance. Mystrom has even spotted a few in his own backyard. Bears are frequent, but less welcome, visitors, too. Flooding of summer lawns, caused by beavers damming streams (and creating watery playgrounds for some 5,000 geese), is viewed as a minor inconvenience.

Many of Anchorage's biggest boosters, including Mystrom, have migrated from places where anything resembling a moose in the backyard would result in an instant 911 call. "I left Los Angeles in the rear view mirror in 1972 and never looked back," says Mystrom, recalling the day he quit his job with toy-maker Mattel, withdrew his savings of $800 from the bank, loaded his wife, Mary, 8-month-old son, Nick, and all their worldly goods in a VW van, and headed north. He first visited Alaska in 1968 while working on a survey crew, and he vowed to return. "Every time I dreamed about the future," he says, "Alaska was there."

A job selling ads for a TV station led to a vice presidency at an advertising agency. Mystrom later bought the agency, in the same year the Alaskan pipeline bill was signed. That changed the state forever. "The economy started booming and so did the agency," he recalls. Mystrom, who sold the company in 1990, admits that all the while he was taking care of business, "the idea of being mayor or governor was always in the back of my mind."

Mystrom warmed up for his current assignment by serving on the city's Municipal Assembly from 1979 to 1985. He also chaired two campaigns to bring the Winter Olympic Games to Anchorage, traveling to 65 countries in the process. Although the Olympics eluded Anchorage, the effort created a lot of good will for the city Mystrom claims is loved by each and every resident.

"People who come here either love it or hate it," Mystrom maintains, matter-of-factly, "and those who hate it tend to leave right away, so I think it's safe to assume that everyone here loves it." They're pretty fond of Mystrom, too, having entrusted the GOP standard-bearer with the keys to city hall in 1994. He's proud of the job he's done—"crime is down, Anchorage is cleaner and prettier, too"—he boasts in the most recent State of the City Report, and he feels his leadership style is appreciated by the voters, most of whom say they're independent, then vote Republican.

Mister Mayor

"I make the distinction between being a manager and a leader," Mystrom explains, uncoiling his lanky frame in a desk chair held together by duct tape in his seventh floor office, "and I'm not a manager. My job is to provide a vision or direction; to develop a strategy for making it happen; to align it—to line up the people to make it happen; then to motivate those people. Those are the only things I should be doing. If I tried to interject myself into the small things, I couldn't do the big things."

Many of the big things on Mystrom's menu take him out of town for long periods of time. Last fall, just before slowing down long enough to be interviewed for this story, his itinerary included jaunts to Memphis, Tennessee, and Louisville, Kentucky, where he pitched the positive aspects of expansion of their Anchorage operations to top management at UPS and FedEx, followed almost immediately by an outing to the Orient.

In Taiwan, Mystrom met with business leaders interested in opening a fish-processing facility in Anchorage. It could eventually employ 400 people. With "tens of millions of salmon" to use as bargaining chips, he was soon on his way to a brainstorming session with a group considering financing modernization of Anchorage's port facilities. Then it was off to the Land of the Rising Sun to encourage Japan Airlines to promote more passenger traffic through Anchorage and to sell some of the city's surplus water.

"When you sell water, or anything else, from Alaska, the marketing is already done," Mystrom maintains. "Asians, in particular, have an image of blue skies, clear water, and sparkling glaciers. Of course, that's all true. The people I was dealing with want to send over fiberglass-lined tankers and buy our water wholesale. I'd prefer to have them open a bottling plant."

Dealing With Diabetes

No matter where he wanders, Mystrom, who found out he had diabetes more than 30 years ago during his undergraduate days at the University of Colorado, keeps a close watch on his glucose readings, checking his blood sugar "five or six times a day." He works in daily doses of exercise, jogging in the morning or taking brisk 5- to 7-mile walks, and working out with weights three times a week. Eating properly on the road can be a challenge, he admits. "With the food being so different, it's hard to predict how many carbohydrates you'll encounter in Japan."

If there's anyone in Anchorage who doesn't know Mystrom has diabetes, it isn't because he's reluctant to talk about it. "I enjoy talking to people just diagnosed, especially young people," Mystrom explains. "I'll get a call from the ADA affiliate office and they'll ask, 'Would you talk with this 10-year-old boy and his mom and dad? He's got diabetes and they don't know what to expect.' Or they might ask me to talk to a guy about my own age who has just been diagnosed and is having a tough time dealing with it."

Mystrom invites his listeners to envision him as he was in 1963—a college sophomore, "pretty athletic, involved in a lot of sports, and hungry all the time." Despite a well-earned reputation for being an eating machine, the future mayor started losing weight, dropping to 150 pounds.

"My roommate talked me into checking with a doctor," Mystrom recalls. "The doctor decided to give me a glucose tolerance test. This was on a Friday. That afternoon I was playing tennis with my girlfriend when my roommate came running across the lawn, yelling that the doctor had called and wanted to see me right away. I remember him saying, 'I think you've got diabetes.' That was the first time I thought about what those words could mean."

The doctor confirmed the roommate's suspicions, gave Mystrom a shot of insulin and some books on diabetes, and suggested that he eat something immediately and come back on Monday with all the questions he was sure to think of over the weekend.

"I went for a long walk by myself, and I remember crying a little bit, being a little scared, and not knowing what was ahead of me in life," Mystrom recalls. "The thought of giving myself a shot every day was really depressing. Then I got this resolve that it wasn't going to happen—that I was going to have such a healthy diet and good lifestyle that I wasn't going to have to take a shot. What I forgot to do was eat. All of a sudden I had my first experience with an insulin reaction."

A quick sprint to a nearby restaurant led to the consumption of an unexceptional hamburger steak that would have long ago been forgotten were it not for one eye-opening fact. "When I finished eating," says Mystrom, "I wasn't hungry for the first time in months. That's when I realized something had really been wrong."

Young Rick returned to the doctor's office the following Monday with "three pages of questions on a yellow legal pad" and a determination not to let diabetes stand in his way. His life-long pursuit of that goal became much easier, he says, when he made the transition to an insulin pump in 1983. "The pump," he proclaims, "is wonderful for traveling."

In addition to sharing his personal story with newly diagnosed patients, Mystrom makes time to participate in Association signature programs (including the Tour de Cure bike ride), and he plans to hold an annual luncheon for city employees who have diabetes. He is also the creator of the Leaders in Innovation Program, which salutes people in Alaska who do new and interesting things. The program includes a presentation about innovations in diabetes research. He wishes he had time to do more.

Michelle Cassano, a fiery former Bostonian who heads the ADA Alaska Affiliate from Anchorage, is one of Mystrom's biggest fans. "I sometimes wonder if Rick realizes the impact he's had," says Michelle. "For years, he was the only well-known businessman in Alaska willing to discuss having diabetes. I've seen him change his schedule on very short notice to go talk with a family who just found out their child had diabetes. He knows how important his personal contact can be."

Personal contact means a lot to Mystrom, who once showed up at an 8 a.m. meeting with visiting business leaders lugging a 65-pound king salmon he'd caught the night before. "I had a reception for them before I went fishing and I told them I'd drop by the next day to let them know how I did," Mystrom says with a smile. "So I brought the fish along with me. I got a big kick out of seeing so many people in suits stumbling all over their charts and graphs so they could get their picture taken with the mayor and his fish."

Mystrom gets such a big kick out of everything associated with being mayor that he probably wishes he could keep the job forever. Unfortunately, the City Charter says the mayor can only serve two consecutive 3-year terms.

Having been bitten by the political bug, and having had half the population of Alaska vote him into office, Mystrom admits that the thought of running for governor still crosses his mind now and then. He just might win. And, as recent history has shown, it isn't impossible for the governor of an obscure state that begins with the letter "A" to end up in the White House. The only glitch in that scenario, to hear Mystrom tell it, is that having dropped anchor in Anchorage for so long, he would find living in Washington pretty dull by comparison.

Roger Doughty is a freelance writer who lives in Minneapolis, Minnesota. He hopes to serve as ambassador to Aruba in a Mystrom administration.

Tony Ciraolo: Making Movie Magic

by Sherrye Landrum

This article appeared in *Diabetes Forecast,* February 1995.

Did you ever know a person who lived in a fantasy world? How about a person who paints one?

Tony Ciraolo is one such artist. But he doesn't confine himself to canvas. He transforms wood and plaster and fabric into stone and sky and rich wood carvings. The fantasy is yours. Your eyes believe the forgery; you do not see his brush strokes.

Tony is a second cousin to the hardworking angels in a William Pene Du Bois children's story who hand paint each animal before it goes to earth. Like those angels, Tony works where we can't see him. And his art becomes "reality" on film.

Tony is a carpenter and a scenic artist who paints movie sets. He's so good at what he does that you don't know where God's blue sky stops and Tony's sky begins. He has fashioned the Alamo from newly cut pine and rendered a Las Vegas hotel lobby more elegant than the real one.

There's No Business Like Show Business

Tony was one of 40 artisans chosen from a group of 3,000 applicants to work on a movie called *Casino,* directed by Martin Scorsese and starring Robert DeNiro, Joe Pesci, James Woods, and Sharon Stone.

When he talks about his work, Tony sounds more proud than starstruck. Working on the set where movie stars perform may sound like a glamorous way to earn a living, but the reality behind the make-believe is long hours and hard work. For everyone. Although his voice gets gravelly with fatigue, Tony shrugs it off saying, "You'll rest when you die. Right?"

He enjoys the work because it's challenging and fun. And a little like living in a cartoon. Especially when he says, "Guess what! Today I made cardboard and wood look like a big metal safe. A car's gonna run through it tomorrow."

For the past 5 years, he's lived in Las Vegas, where he's earned laurels as a master carpenter. Drawing on his "movie" skills, he's built elaborate sets for entertainers such as Siegfried and Roy (who have a famous magic and white tiger act), but he's also helped build real houses and world-class hotels.

Tony made his set-painter name in California at the Lorimar studios before he moved to Las Vegas. He worked on several television series there, including *Dallas* and *Knots Landing.* He was behind the scenes for Dodge, Diet Coke, and Pepsi commercials, and for the animated film *Beauty and the Beast.* After his work on Michael Jackson's video for the hit song "The Way You Make Me Feel," Jackson's director's chair came home with him.

A Family Affair

Tony may have inherited a considerable portion of his talent. His father was a well-known and respected scenic artist in Hollywood. "Sure he was," says Tony, with obvious pride. "He ran the back-lot art department at Universal Studios for years." You may have seen his work—but didn't know you did—in such films as *Earthquake, The Ten Commandments,* and *Planet of the Apes.* Tony's brother, Joey, is also a set painter of renown with 18 years experience. Among the movies he's "painted" are *The Terminator, Terminator 2, Die Hard, Die Hard 2,* and *Hoffa.* It seems pretty clear that in the wonderful world backstage at the movies, the name Ciraolo will get you in the door—particularly if you have a paintbrush in your hand.

"I make new things look old," says Tony, describing work he recently did on a set of the Alamo. "I took new wood and aged it 200 years." The art director, seeing the quality of this work, nodded and said, "Yes, you are your father's son."

Making movie magic is a theme that shows up else-where in Tony's family. His mother did casting for a long time before his father died. His little sister, Peach, an accountant for a "funny safe" company (they make safes disguised as common household objects such as a can of soup), is married to a prop man for the television series *Coach*. His brother's girlfriend won an Academy Award for Best Make-up Artist for her work on Robin Williams' *Mrs. Doubtfire*.

But no matter who they share scenes with, Tony's family remains a down-to-earth, loving Italian family. Laurie, Joey, Tony, Donna, and Peach. "In my father's eyes," says Tony, "we could never do wrong." And his mother, Marie, says her children are "very, very close-knit. They're always hugging. It's the first thing everyone notices about them."

Mr. Personality

Tony, 33, doesn't seem to have suffered from being the middle child. In front of or behind the scenes—he's a scene stealer. He's a wise guy. He's a sweetheart. He's a clown. He's generous with his good humor—and like anyone who succeeds in show business, he tries to always leave 'em smiling.

It would be difficult to say if the diabetes that he developed when he was 8 years old helped shape his irrepressible good spirits, but diabetes certainly never dampened those spirits for long.

In Tony's philosophy, what happens to you is not as important as how you look at it. Tony prefers to look at almost everything through eyes crinkled with laughter. And when he's not clowning around, he says simply, "Because of diabetes, I know I can handle anything." And most people agree with him.

He took diabetes in stride as a boy. He says, "Hey, my doctor told me, 'Tony, this is your disease. You have to learn to handle it yourself.' So I did." Diabetes became just another part of Tony being Tony. He was never afraid of what his body needed. He and his mom even taught his friends to give insulin shots. "Sure, everybody got a shot at Tony," he says with a laugh. "Why not?"

In fact, all the neighborhood friends (who are still

close) carried sugar cubes for Tony on their camping trips and knew not to drink the Cokes because they were Tony's.

His mom is warm and supportive and as good-humored as Tony. It's easy to see they share an outlook on life. When she helped organize the first bike-a-thon in California to raise funds for diabetes research, she didn't know that someday she would develop type 2 diabetes. She and Tony are the only ones in the family with diabetes.

Half The Battle Is Knowing What You Like

Tony is a man who enjoys life. Diabetes has not kept him from a challenging and varied career. Nor has it stopped him from being an enthusiastic athlete. He has three favorite windsurf boards and a well-used bicycle. He remembers once having a hypoglycemic reaction standing in line waiting for a ski lift. He passed out, but this hasn't kept him off of the slopes.

Why? Because Tony is serious about one thing—keeping active and healthy. His heart's been captured by the physical thrill of windsurfing. He takes long bike rides. And he readily admits to stopping off at a glitzy Las Vegas hotel if he needs a soda to bring his blood glucose back up. Through sports, he has learned to listen to his body, and this helps him keep the diabetes under control.

He carries fruit juice and fruit with him when he goes windsurfing in case of low blood glucose. And he says he deals with long hours and erratic eating on the set by "taking his lunch."

The Test

This comfort zone with his diabetes has helped him through the toughest test of his "I-can-handle-anything" attitude. In February 1990, a bad car wreck crushed both of his legs. The surgeons surveyed the massive damage and assumed that he would not heal because of his diabetes. They decided to amputate both legs.

Tony argued passionately that they try to repair them instead. Even in the emergency room, he presented his case with humor. "If you have to cut something, take this beard. I don't need it."

Like Gus McCrae in *Lonesome Dove,* Tony needed his legs in order to be Tony. He didn't want to kick any pigs (Gus's reason for keeping his), but he did want to windsurf and paint and be a carpenter. Climbing around a movie set would probably be impossible without legs. Tony simply could not let them go.

Reluctantly, the surgeons agreed to try to save his legs. At the time, neither they nor Tony had any idea that it would take 3½ years and 30 surgeries before his legs would heal. Tony says, "I was only awake on Tuesdays and Thursdays. The rest of the time I was in the operating room."

It was not diabetes that made it difficult for him to heal. He developed osteomyelitis, an infection of the bone and the bone marrow. Dee Riley, RN, the home health nurse who changed his dressings and cared for him for a year, says, "This condition is rarely cured. Cleaning out the infection left wounds right down to the bone, which even for a nurse are quite intimidating. At the hospital, they sent him up to the burn unit to have the dressings changed." But Tony kept coming home.

After a few months, Riley and the other nurse who shared Tony's care were telling him, "You're crazy. Just give up." But he wouldn't, and she says his healing is "more than amazing—beyond amazing! He has such an incredible drive that nothing really slows him down."

The Cage

Tony's recovery involved thousands of prayers and several miracles, including an external fixator device invented by a Russian country doctor, G.S. Ilizarov, called the "cage." The cage, an elaborate birdcage of wires threaded through the muscles and bones of his legs, held the pieces of bone together while they healed. (For more about this time in Tony's life, see *Diabetes Forecast,* November 1991, Celebrating Life, pp. 76–77.)

The cages were very painful, but he had them on for so long, they became part of his life. After 3 years of waiting to get back on the water, he even went windsurfing with one still on—just as soon as his doctor approved it!

Another miracle was Tony's attitude. The doctors and nurses who helped him heal marveled at that. He kept his part of the bargain—faith, hope, and good humor—through the weeks and months and years of pain and difficult surgeries and not being able to work. His mother says, "Out of all my kids, only Tony could do it. It's his determination." Tony's staunch refusal to let go of his sense of humor and his legs may be the reason he's walking today.

Tony credits his family—for whom the drive from California to Las Vegas became a standard weekend activity—and his friends, especially former fiancee Susie Robson and his roommate Vic Casimero, with helping him keep his spirits up.

At his sister's wedding in October, Tony escorted his mother down the aisle. Family friends, many of whom have known Tony all his life, looked on with tears in their eyes. This amazing young man continues to celebrate life, and he walks without a limp.

Making It Up As He Went Along

No medical textbook addresses controlling diabetes through trauma as extreme as Tony's. So while the doctors devised ways to put his legs back together, he figured out how to keep his blood glucose levels normal.

Pain, stress, anesthesia, medications, and enforced bed rest—all are part of surgery and all affect blood glucose levels. Most people have to prepare for surgery once or twice in their lives. For Tony, it was a weekly event. He says, "For what it took to monitor my insulin, food, and drug intake through all this, I could be a chemist!"

"He's exceptionally in tune with his body and does an exceptional job at keeping his blood glucose in the normal range," says Riley. At each visit they played a guessing game—Tony would tell her what his blood glucose was before he tested. He was always within 10 points of his real blood glucose level. "He has," she adds, "a little computer in his head. He just knows what he needs."

A bout of retinopathy added to his pain 2 years into the process, but his eyes responded well to laser surgery. He's proven his claim. After all this, he's pretty sure he can handle anything.

Four and a half years after the crash, as he walks around the set and renews old acquaintances, those who knew him before the accident are amazed. And happy to see him.

"Yes, Tony's back," he says, and happiness warms the last of the tiredness right out of his voice. "I got my legs back. I'm surfing again. It's 'have tools, will travel' time for me. Every day above ground is a good one."

Sherrye Landrum is a book editor at ADA and a former departments editor for Diabetes Forecast.

Eva Saxl: A Remarkable Life

by Marcia Levine Mazur

This article appeared in *Diabetes Forecast,* July 1991.

This is a tale of heroism and survival, a saga of adventure and endurance that spans four continents. But mostly, this is a love story that has lasted more than 50 years.

It revolves around Eva Saxl, who received the American Diabetes Association's Charles H. Best Medal for Distinguished Service in the Cause of Diabetes at the International Diabetes Federation Congress in Washington, D.C., on June 25, 1991.

Saxl's story began more than 57 years ago in Prague, Czechoslovakia, when 13-year-old Eva told her mother she would marry no one but her distant relative Victor Saxl.

Eva, the daughter of a wealthy Jewish family, attended finishing schools in England and Switzerland, and spoke seven languages by the time she was 16. Because she had poor eyesight, her parents provided her with a special maid, and she lived in a world of culture and refinement. Then came 1939 and the Nazi invasion of Czechoslovakia that shattered that world forever.

Still, on February 15, 1940—at age 19—Eva married her Victor. Barely 3 months later, the newlyweds fled, knowing they were leaving country and family forever. They carried only a few articles of clothing and 20 deutschmarks between them—about $2—the maximum the Nazis allowed.

The pair made it to Italy, and, as World War II ignited Europe, they boarded the last ship to escape through the Suez Canal. It was headed for one of the few countries that accepted Jews escaping Nazi persecution—China. However, escape was expensive. Their entry visas for China had cost thousands.

The Saxls made their home in Shanghai, and things went well at first. Victor became manager of the largest woolen mill in China, and Eva—already studying Chinese aboard ship—taught languages. But then she began losing weight and feeling insatiably thirsty.

The Sugar Water Disease

The doctor gave his diagnosis in Chinese, but Eva understood both the words—"it's the sugar water disease"—and their meaning—diabetes.

Though unhappy about the diagnosis, Eva was not really worried. Insulin was readily available, she was doing well, and, of course, she had Victor. He promised he would take care of her. "His love helped me avoid the psychological problems of diabetes," she recalls.

Then came December 7, 1941, and the Japanese surprise attack on Pearl Harbor. One day later, the Japanese marched into Shanghai and issued orders to close the pharmacies. People with diabetes rushed through the city buying all the insulin they could find, but it wasn't long before there was no more available—legally.

After that, only crisp new U.S. dollars—many of them—or gold bars could buy the insulin on the black market, quality unknown. Eva recalls Teng, a friend who took black market insulin. He died after one injection; the insulin was contaminated.

As the supply dwindled, people with type 1 diabetes sickened; some died. Those left began a near-starvation diet, so their bodies would require less of their precious store. Eva, like others, tried replacing insulin with Chinese herbs and other medications. Nothing worked.

To keep Eva from worrying about how low her supply was, Victor secretly refilled old insulin bottles with water and milk powder.

"He Loved Me."

Actually, though, Victor was desperate. He had promised to take care of his Eva, and she needed insulin. She put it simply. "He loved me. He didn't want me to die." To save his wife, and the others with diabetes in Shanghai,

Victor begged local physicians: Help me make insulin. Although they refused to get involved, they lent him their medical books—in six languages.

Victor, a textile engineer, knew only textile chemistry, but one book had drawings and a clear description of how Banting and Best, discoverers of insulin, had done their work.

Victor located a Chinese chemist, Mr. Wong, who volunteered his primitive laboratory. To get the pancreases needed for insulin production, Eva and their cook, Chi Ching, would ride out to a slaughterhouse at 5 a.m. and claim the pancreases from newly killed large animals, mainly water buffalo and pigs. They'd stuff the fresh pancreases into a wide-mouth flask and rush it by rickshaw to the laboratory. There, Eva could grind it in the meat grinder.

Victor's experiments progressed slowly, while Eva's stock of insulin dwindled fast. Everything took time, including testing the new insulin on rabbits, first to see if the rabbits lived, and then to figure the insulin's strength.

Finally, when only a 5-day supply remained, Victor arrived home with a bottle of brown liquid. To keep Eva from worrying, he told her it was Japanese insulin made from fish—and she pretended to believe him. But both knew the truth; this was the insulin Victor had made. And both understood that—although it had been tested on rabbits—no one knew its effect on humans. This injection was an experiment.

After telling Eva the "fish insulin" might cause pain, Victor injected it, then his eyes filled with tears. He told her to pray, and even had her take a sedative to help get through the stress. But it didn't take long before they knew. The insulin worked! "We were crazy with happiness," Eva recalled.

Not One Died

People signed up for the insulin, and helped with money and supplies, but those were tough years for the more than 400 people with diabetes in the small Shanghai community. There was never enough ice and alcohol for the production, and Victor discovered that ordinary bottles harmed the insulin. Fortunately, those who used insulin had held onto their old bottles, a link with the old days, when those bottles had held what they now desperately needed.

Batches of the brown insulin were small, and only half of the supply was acceptable. Electricity might fail and disrupt the work, and, toward the end, there were Allied bombings to contend with. But insulin distribution went strictly according to the list.

Although some who needed insulin died before Victor's insulin production began, no one died afterwards.

Three years later, in 1945, the city was liberated, and the Saxls faced yet another problem. There was little future for them in China; Europe was in ruin; it was extremely difficult for immigrants to enter countries like the United States; and there was no State of Israel to accept Jewish refugees. They didn't know where to turn. Then President Truman signed a bill allowing people with special abilities to emigrate to the U.S., and Eva and Victor qualified.

They sailed into San Francisco Bay aboard an American troop ship. In California, Eva asked every drugstore if they had insulin, amazed at how ordinary a commodity it was here.

Hello To Harry

On the ship, Marines had told the Saxls to see America before settling down. So, they took a train across the United States, stopping at famous sights and cities.

In Independence, Missouri, they knocked on President Truman's door. "We wanted to thank Mr. Truman for letting us into America," Eva explained. "He said no one else had ever done that." The Trumans invited them to tea. "We had a marvelous time," she remembered. He also gave them a letter to a friend of his—international financier Bernard Baruch.

After their visit with the Trumans, Eva and Victor continued their trip across the country, and settled on the East Coast. They became U.S. citizens and Eva was always "a proud American."

One of their first priorities was to get medical attention for Eva, so they visited a diabetes specialist in New York. That visit became another milestone in their lives.

In the doctor's office, Victor set a bottle of the brown insulin from Shanghai on the desk; the doctor thought it was urine. "When we explained that it was insulin Victor had made, he nearly fell off his chair," Eva laughed. The doctor contacted the American Diabetes Association, and the Association asked Eva and Victor to tour the country, talking about their Shanghai years.

News of their remarkable achievements spread, and in 1952 they met Charles Best, co-discoverer of insulin. He invited them to speak at a roundtable in Toronto, the city where he and Frederick Banting had discovered insulin. "Dr. Best really appreciated what Victor had done, and he wanted all the details of our story," Eva recalled. The pair accepted Dr. Best's invitation to tour Canada and tell of their experiences.

The same year, they met pioneer diabetes researcher Elliot P. Joslin, then 82, who taught Eva about diabetes care and lent her books on the subject.

The producers of radio and the new medium of television were intrigued by the Saxl's story, and Eva and Victor appeared on a number of radio and TV shows. Even Hollywood took note as the Hal Roach Studios retold the story of the brown insulin in a TV documentary.

Victor Brought Me Here

In 1968, Victor, who had been working for a large textile firm in New York, took a position with the United Nations Technical Assistance Board (now called UNIDO).

The United Nations sent the couple to South America. On their third day in Santiago, Chile, Victor suffered a sudden heart attack and died. Eva was grief stricken.

She stayed on in Chile, although she retained her U.S. citizenship and returned to the United States every 2 years for medical checkups. Still, she felt at home in Chile because her only brother had settled there. "And," she said, "Victor brought me here."

Eva never regretted the decision. At the age of 71 when she received the ADA award, Eva, whose eye problems were not diabetes related, was considered legally blind. But she continued to work for the advancement of diabetes care under the auspices of a number of Chilean organizations. She was particularly concerned about the children of Chile.

Eva was one of the organizers of the Foundacion Diabetes Juvenil de Chile, which now has 882 members with type 1 diabetes. Vivian Rojas, editor of Chile's *Diabetes Control* magazine, said, "In our process of becoming strong to help others, Eva played an important role with her expertise, personal experience, and charm."

Eva attended meetings around the world helping spread the word on diabetes care. She found one invitation particularly dramatic, and she was pleased to accept. It was an invitation to be guest of honor and speaker at the German Diabetes Association Congress in Dusseldorf.

She was also invited back to her native Prague, where she was made first member of honor of the Czechoslovakia Parents and Friends of Diabetic Children. In Prague, she visited her old neighborhood. "But without loved ones, it's not the same," she said.

Eva's honors include the prestigious FAND-MILES award from the International Diabetes Federation for her work in diabetes education in developing nations and the Achievement Award for Living Well with Diabetes from the International Diabetes Center in Minneapolis.

In 1966 she was presented with the Joslin Diabetes Center's Quarter Century Victory Medal for patients who remain free of diabetic complications after 25 years on insulin. In 1991, she was awarded the Joslin 50-Year Medal.

Eva continued to be in good health. "I am not a saint, but I eat rather carefully," she said. She had no major complications, although she said, "I have had some nasty hypoglycemic reactions off-and-on for 50 years."

Her philosophy was always upbeat and optimistic. "I feel that whatever I went through was just something that had to be coped with in a way that would help others."

Like most satisfying love stories, this one has a happy ending, in its way. In her essay in Edward R. Murrow's book *This I Believe,* Eva wrote, "Besides my trust in God, I derived the greatest strength from the deep love and complete understanding between my husband and me."

She continued to derive strength from that love all her life.

Marcia Levine Mazur is senior editor of Diabetes Forecast.

About the American Diabetes Association

The American Diabetes Association is the nation's leading voluntary health organization supporting diabetes research, information, and advocacy. Founded in 1940, the Association provides services to communities across the country. Its mission is to prevent and cure diabetes and to improve the lives of all people affected by diabetes.

For more than 50 years, the American Diabetes Association has been the leading publisher of comprehensive diabetes information for people with diabetes and the health care professionals who treat them. Its huge library of practical and authoritative books for people with diabetes covers every aspect of self care—cooking and nutrition, fitness, weight control, medications, complications, emotional issues, and general self care. The Association also publishes books and medical treatment guides for physicians and other health care professionals.

Membership in the Association is available to health care professionals and people with diabetes and includes subscriptions to one or more of the Association's periodicals. People with diabetes receive *Diabetes Forecast,* the nation's leading health and wellness magazine for people with diabetes. Health care professionals receive one or more of the Association's five scientific and medical journals.

For more information, please call toll-free:

Questions about diabetes:	1-800-DIABETES
Membership, people with diabetes:	1-800-806-7801
Membership, health professionals:	1-800-232-3472
Free catalog of ADA books:	1-800-232-6733
Visit us on the Web:	www.diabetes.org
Visit us at our Web bookstore:	www.diabetes.store